What Do I Eat Now?

A Step-by-Step Guide to Eating
Right with Type 2 Diabetes 2nd Edition

Tami A. Ross, RDN, LD, CDE, MLDE, and
Patti B. Geil, MS, RDN, CDE, MLDE, FAND, FAADE

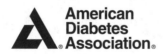

American
Diabetes
Association®

Director, Book Publishing, Abe Ogden; *Managing Editor,* Greg Guthrie; *Acquisitions Editor,* Victor Van Beuren; *Project Manager,* Boldface LLC; *Production Manager,* Melissa Sprott; *Composition,* Circle Graphics; *Cover Design,* Vis-à-Vis Creative Concepts; *Printer,* Versa Press.

Printed in the United States of America
3 5 7 9 10 8 6 4 2

The suggestions and information contained in this publication are generally consistent with the *Standards of Medical Care in Diabetes* and other policies of the American Diabetes Association, but they do not represent the policy or position of the Association or any of its boards or committees. Reasonable steps have been taken to ensure the accuracy of the information presented. However, the American Diabetes Association cannot ensure the safety or efficacy of any product or service described in this publication. Individuals are advised to consult a physician or other appropriate health care professional before undertaking any diet or exercise program or taking any medication referred to in this publication. Professionals must use and apply their own professional judgment, experience, and training and should not rely solely on the information contained in this publication before prescribing any diet, exercise, or medication. The American Diabetes Association—its officers, directors, employees, volunteers, and members—assumes no responsibility or liability for personal or other injury, loss, or damage that may result from the suggestions or information in this publication.

Dr. Maria Mupanomunda conducted the internal review of this book to ensure that it meets American Diabetes Association guidelines.

♾ The paper in this publication meets the requirements of the ANSI Standard Z39.48-1992 (permanence of paper).

American Diabetes Association titles may be purchased for business or promotional use or for special sales. To purchase more than 50 copies of this book at a discount, or for custom editions of this book with your logo, contact the American Diabetes Association at the address below or at booksales@diabetes.org.

American Diabetes Association
1701 North Beauregard Street
Alexandria, Virginia 22311

DOI: 10.2337/9781580405584

Library of Congress Cataloging-in-Publication Data

Ross, Tami, author.
  What do I eat now? : a step-by-step guide to eating right with Type 2 diabetes / Tami A. Ross, RDN, LD, CDE, MLDE & Patti B. Geil, MS, RDN, CDE, MLDE, FAND, FAADE. — Second edition.
    pages cm
  Revision of: What do I eat now? / Patti B. Geil & Tami A. Ross.
  Includes index.
  Summary: "This book will help the reader simplify life with diabetes by leading them through basic nutrition survival skills and behavior changes. Food and nutrition options are clearly outlined, and specific meal menus with simple, wholesome recipes are given" — Provided by publisher.
  ISBN 978-1-58040-558-4 (paperback)
  1. Diabetes—Diet therapy—Recipes. 2. Diabetics—Nutrition. I. Geil, Patti Bazel, author. II. Title.
  RC662.G452 2015
  641.5'6314—dc23
                          2015011143

To all of my patients over the years who have said, "Just tell me what to eat!": Thank you. You are the inspiration for this book.

T.A.R.

To those who face the challenge of healthy eating while living with diabetes every day: You can do it! Remember, there is no diet that will do what healthy eating does.

Skip the diet. Just eat healthy.

P.B.G.

Change for the Better!

Perhaps you've just been diagnosed with type 2 diabetes. Or maybe you've had diabetes for some time and haven't been able to control your blood glucose levels to the degree that you'd like. Whether you are newly diagnosed or have a newfound interest in diabetes self-management, you'll discover that healthy eating is fundamental to taking good care of yourself.

Managing type 2 diabetes can feel like an overwhelming challenge at times. Research has shown that if an individual with type 2 diabetes who takes an oral medication followed all of the standard recommendations for self-care, it would consume 143 minutes of each day. Those two or more hours spent each day checking blood glucose levels, taking medication, exercising, and eating right translate into a part-time job! Even more, it probably wouldn't surprise you to find out that of the 143 minutes required to care for your diabetes, almost half of them would be related to food: meal planning, shopping, and preparing meals. Add to this the often conflicting nutrition advice you hear from friends and the media. It's enough to make you throw up your hands in frustration and shout, "Can't somebody just tell me what to eat?"

How This Book Can Help

What Do I Eat Now? has been written to help simplify your life with diabetes by leading you through basic nutrition survival skills and behavior changes. Your food and nutrition options are clearly outlined, and you will be given specific meal menus with simple, wholesome recipes. At the same time, you will learn about a diabetes nutrition topic in each chapter and see the next steps you need to take to reach your goal of healthier eating. Over time, the lessons you learn can help you make the right food decisions in whatever situations you may face, from eating out, to surviving holidays, to enjoying favorite family recipes. We routinely hear from our patients that making those "better-for-you" food decisions soon becomes habit.

Each chapter of *What Do I Eat Now?* contains:

- **A menu for breakfast, lunch, dinner, snack time, or a special occasion.** The menus provide you with two options: a meal of 45–60 grams of carbohydrate, or one with 60–75 grams of carbohydrate. You can choose the option that best meets your individual nutrition needs. You'll also find tips for making each menu simpler and quicker. If grams of carbohydrate are new to you, an explanation will follow in Chapter 2.
- **A recipe from that chapter's menu, complete with nutrition analysis.** By the time you finish this book, you'll have many quick, easy, and delicious recipes to add to your personal collection.

Remember, the best nutrition plan is one that's individualized based on your food preferences to help you achieve optimal diabetes control and overall health. Work with your registered dietitan/registered dietitian nutritionist (RD/RDN) and diabetes health-care team to determine which menus, recipes, and tips are right for you.

Preparation Is the Secret to Success

The first step to achieving success in following a healthy meal plan for diabetes is to visualize what that success looks like for you.

- How do you see yourself managing your meal plan a month from now?
- Will you be eating breakfast every morning?
- Will you have replaced your mid-afternoon run to the vending machine with a healthy snack from home?
- Will you be making better choices in the grocery store, based on what you read on food labels?

Take the first step by imagining where you would like to be a month from now, and then start making plans to learn and do what you need to do to make your vision a reality.

Setting Goals and Taking Action

As you work through this book, you will be making great strides! The first step to moving forward is to set goals for your nutrition plan over the next month. Your diabetes management will have new meaning when you set goals and go after them with enthusiasm. Of course, you might not accomplish every goal you set; nearly no one does. But having goals and striving to reach them is what really matters.

Setting goals sounds like a big job, but S.M.A.R.T. goal setting gives you a framework for getting it done, as well as a better chance of succeeding at your goals. "S.M.A.R.T." is an acronym for Specific, Measurable, Achievable, Realistic, and Time Bound, the 5 qualities that you should aim for when setting goals. Create an action plan for results by setting goals that are:

SPECIFIC: A specific goal has a greater chance of being achieved.

MEASURABLE: Measuring progress keeps you on track.

ACHIEVABLE: An achievable goal is tied to small, easily accomplished steps.

REALISTIC: A realistic goal is one you are willing and able to work toward.

TIME BOUND: A time frame gives you a sense of urgency.

Here are a few imprecise diabetes nutrition goals, translated into S.M.A.R.T. format:

Initial goal	S.M.A.R.T. goal
"I will eat more fruits and vegetables."	"I will have a medium fresh orange for breakfast three days this week."
"I will eat healthier on the road."	"I will order a side salad instead of french fries at lunch five days a week and have the dressing on the side."
"I will choose better snacks."	"I will eat a snack of whole-grain crackers and low-fat cheese from home instead of going to the vending machine every afternoon at work."

Behavior Is What You Do, Not What You Know

Diabetes is unlike other medical conditions in one important way: individuals with diabetes manage their own condition 95% of the time. It's not possible or practical for you to ask for medical advice every time you plan to eat, take your medication, or deal with a minor illness. When you walk out of your diabetes health-care team's office, you are the one who will make the day-to-day decisions about your diabetes care. Of course, you will have a team of health professionals available as needed, but ultimately, the responsibility for your diabetes care rests with you.

To be a successful self-manager and enjoy good health and well-being, you need to know the facts about managing your diabetes, specifically, your blood glucose goals, how much carbohydrate you should eat, and the type and amount of physical activity you need each day. This knowledge can be gained through sessions with your diabetes healthcare team and from the many resources available to you in print and online. However, knowing what you need to do and actually doing it are two very different things. For instance, after consulting with your healthcare team, you may know that you personally should walk at least 30 minutes every day, but maybe you can't seem to find the time. Or you know you've been advised to check your blood glucose at least twice each day, but sticking your finger is not fun, so you avoid it. And you know that third piece of pizza will send your blood glucose skyrocketing, but it just tastes so good. How many times have you said, "I know what I should do, but I just can't seem to do it?"

Over the years, diabetes health professionals have come to realize that, in addition to providing education, helping individuals with diabetes change their behavior is the key to successful diabetes self-management. Much research has been done in the area of behavior change. While working in the area of addiction, professor of psychology Dr. James Prochaska and colleagues developed the "Transtheoretical Model of Change" as a way of explaining why certain individuals were able to change poor habits, while others were "stuck" and unable to adopt healthier actions. According to Prochaska's "Stages of Change" model, people are in different stages regarding their readiness to adopt a healthy behavior or stop an unhealthy one, and this affects their ability to change. These stages of change are:

- Precontemplation
- Contemplation
- Preparation
- Action
- Maintenance

Prochaska's work has been translated into the area of diabetes self-management education, helping health professionals match their education efforts and advice to the needs of the specific individual with diabetes at any one time, no matter which stage of change that individual currently occupies. **On the next page you'll find some examples of how the stages of change might apply to someone with type 2 diabetes who is overweight.**

Stage of change	Characteristics	Weight-loss example
Precontemplation	Unaware that change is needed or having no intention of changing.	"I feel fine, even though I might be a few pounds overweight."
Contemplation	Intends to change in the next 6 months; aware of the benefits and costs of change.	"I will try to lose some weight. It will help improve my blood glucose. But I don't know if I can give up my wife's home cooking."
Preparation	Ready to change in the next 30 days; taking steps to begin making a change.	"I've looked at all the diets out there. I think I'll stick with the meal plan the registered dietitian nutritionist made with me at my last visit."
Action	Has been making changes within the past 6 months.	"I've been following my meal plan and weighing myself every week for the past month."
Maintenance	Has successfully made a change for more than 6 months; making efforts to avoid slipping into past behaviors.	"Since the holidays are coming up, I need to plan on sticking with my current strategies, so I won't gain weight again this year."

Although you might progress through the stages of change in an orderly fashion, change doesn't always come smoothly. At times, you may move one stage forward then two stages back, but you can learn from your mistakes and use them to move forward again. For example, let's say you began a weight-loss program at the first of the year, but due to stress at home and on the job, you've gone back to your old ways of eating and just can't find the energy to start your meal plan again. Suddenly, you've moved from "action" back to "precontemplation."

The important thing is to learn some healthy ways to cope with stress and move back into "action" again.

As you think about your own diabetes situation, you might find that you're in a different stage of change for each area of diabetes management. For example, you could be in the "maintenance" stage for physical activity because you've been walking 10,000 steps three times a week for the past year. However, you might still be in the "contemplation" stage regarding blood glucose monitoring because you are just beginning to realize the benefits that knowing your numbers could add to your diabetes management.

Where Are You in the Stages of Behavior Change?

Below are a few important areas of diabetes self-management. Where are you in the stages of behavior change for each one?

Diabetes task	Your stage of change
Eating healthy	
Participating in regular physical activity	
Checking your blood glucose	
Taking your medication	

Take a moment to congratulate yourself on those behavior changes you've successfully accomplished! And for those areas that might still need work, think about the benefits and costs of making progress on them. If you decide that now is the time to jump into action, take the first step by calling your diabetes health-care team and asking for the help you need. They will be pleased to assist you in moving toward better diabetes self-management!

Here's to Successful Self-Management!

It's been said that a goal without a plan is just a wish. As you move through each chapter of *What Do I Eat Now?*, you will be guided in making nutrition goals and specific action plans, and you will discover a variety of menus and recipes that you may enjoy and that can work for you. Remember, you are the manager of your diabetes. Let's start on the road to good nutrition by taking the next step to successful self-management!

Take a moment to jot down your goals under "Next Steps." Keep them where you can look at them often. We'll be revisiting your goals in Chapter 11 so you can celebrate what you've accomplished.

Of course, you can't accomplish all of your goals at once. Prioritize the goals that are important to you. Which one will you work on first? Which will have the most impact on your health? Listing your goals in order of importance and then starting with only the first goal on the list will focus your efforts, help you feel less overwhelmed, and reward you with a sense of accomplishment.

Next Steps

Set three S.M.A.R.T. goals for improving your diabetes nutrition and then prioritize them.

My S.M.A.R.T. goals are:

1. _____
   _____

2. _____
   _____

3. _____
   _____

I will work on my goals in this order:

1. _____
   _____

2. _____
   _____

3. _____
   _____

Today is the first day of your journey to good health and well-being with a top-notch diabetes nutrition plan. As you learned in the Introduction, the majority of diabetes care is self-care. Managing your nutrition when you have diabetes involves learning as much as you can about your condition as well as making positive behavior changes related to food. It's time to get started learning about diabetes and its relationship to food. Welcome to Diabetes and Nutrition 101!

Even if you've just been diagnosed with type 2 diabetes, you may be surprised to find that you could have had diabetes for quite some time. This is because type 2 diabetes usually develops gradually, and its symptoms can be so subtle that they may go unnoticed for a while. Looking back, you might realize that you had some of these classic diabetes symptoms even before you were diagnosed:

- Urinating often
- Feeling very thirsty
- Feeling very hungry
- Unusual fatigue
- Blurry vision
- Cuts and bruises that are slow to heal
- Unexplained weight loss
- Tingling, pain, or numbness in your hands or feet
- Dry or itchy skin
- Recurring infections

Many people ignore these symptoms or simply chalk them up to "getting older." Then they put off visiting their health-care provider because the symptoms don't seem serious, which further delays the diabetes diagnosis.

If you have already been diagnosed with type 2 diabetes, then you may know that your family could also have an increased risk for the condition. Fortunately, the same healthy eating and physical activity plan that you will be following can give your family members a better chance at delaying or preventing type 2 diabetes if they join you in your journey toward health and well-being.

What Is Type 2 Diabetes? Can It Be Prevented?

Type 2 diabetes is a lifelong condition marked by high levels of glucose (sugar) in the blood. It begins when the body does not respond correctly to insulin, which is a hormone released by the pancreas. Insulin allows glucose to move into cells, so the glucose can be used for energy. If glucose doesn't get into the cells, then it will build up in the bloodstream, causing the symptoms of diabetes.

Insulin resistance and obesity are usually associated with type 2 diabetes. Insulin resistance means that fat, liver, and muscle cells do not respond normally to insulin, and, as a result, the pancreas produces more and more insulin. But over time it isn't able to keep up. Eventually, the pancreas cannot produce enough insulin to cover the increased needs, and then blood glucose levels rise. The diagnosis of prediabetes or diabetes is based on the results of blood glucose testing. (More information on prediabetes follows.)

Type 2 diabetes is a progressive condition that develops in a predictable pattern. Over time, the body's insulin-producing cells gradually lose their ability to function well, and treatments such as oral medications, injectable medications, or both may be needed—in addition to healthy eating, physical activity, and behavior change—to maintain the best blood glucose control.

The good news is that the progressive nature of type 2 diabetes often allows you or your health-care professional to recognize the developing condition in its early stage, known as prediabetes. Making simple lifestyle changes at the point of prediabetes can prevent or delay the development of type 2 diabetes.

According to the *National Diabetes Statistic Report, 2014,** over 29 million Americans had diabetes in 2014—mainly type 2 diabetes—and over 8 million of those people are not even aware that they have it!

*Available at www.cdc.gov/diabetes/data/statistics/2014statisticsreport.html

What Do the Numbers Mean?

Diagnosis	Fasting blood glucose level	Two-hour glucose on oral glucose tolerance test	A1C
Normal blood glucose	<100 mg/dL	<140 mg/dL	<5.7%
Prediabetes	100–125 mg/dL	140–199 mg/dL	5.7–6.4%
Diabetes	≥126 mg/dL	≥200 mg/dL	≥6.5%

Here are a few things you need to know about glucose testing:

- A fasting blood glucose level is taken when you've had nothing to eat or drink, except water, for 8 hours before the test.
- A 2-hour oral glucose tolerance test is a special test during which you are given a glucose drink and your blood glucose levels are checked 2 hours later.
- The A1C test, which doesn't require fasting or a glucose drink, measures your average blood glucose for the past 2–3 months.
- Diabetes can also be diagnosed using a random (sometimes called "casual") blood glucose test, taken at any time of day. It is often used when you are showing classic diabetes symptoms. Diabetes is diagnosed when a random blood glucose level is ≥200 mg/dL.

Prediabetes: How Diabetes Develops

Prediabetes is the first step in the development of type 2 diabetes. In people with prediabetes, blood glucose levels are above the normal range but below the level at which diabetes is diagnosed. **Prediabetes is diagnosed when:**

- Fasting blood glucose is between 100 mg/dL and 125 mg/dL

- OR the 2-hour glucose value on an oral glucose tolerance test is between 140 mg/dL and 199 mg/dL
- OR the A1C test is between 5.7% and 6.4%

Many people with prediabetes develop type 2 diabetes within 10 years. There are about 86 million people aged 20 years and older with prediabetes in the U.S. If you have prediabetes, then you will be happy to know

Energy Balance Is Important in Delaying or Preventing Type 2 Diabetes

Balancing energy intake (calories from food and beverages) with energy expenditure (through physical activity) leads to weight maintenance.

Achieving weight loss or weight gain means altering the balance between energy intake and energy expenditure. The energy intake (number of calories) you need is based on your age, gender, height, weight, and physical activity.

Since insulin resistance associated with prediabetes and type 2 diabetes is reduced by weight loss, many individuals find they could benefit from dropping a few pounds. To get an idea of your calorie needs until you can meet with a registered dietitan (RD)/registered dietitian nutritionist (RDN), you may find one of these resources helpful:

- **SuperTracker (available at www.supertracker.usda.gov)**—this online tool helps you track what you currently eat and drink, gives you a personalized plan for what you should eat and drink, and guides you to make better nutrition choices.
- **MyFitnessPal (available at www.myfitnesspal.com)**—this is a free, easy-to-use calorie counter.

that it is a condition that responds well to healthy eating habits, weight loss, and exercise. A very large research study called the Diabetes Prevention Program (which included a nutrition counseling component) found that modest weight loss (about 7% of your body weight) and physical activity (at least 30 minutes a day of moderate-intensity activity, five days a week) reduced the chances of prediabetes developing into diabetes by 58%. Lifestyle changes provided even better results than treating prediabetes with medication! Although some health-care professionals may recommend a medication to prevent type 2 diabetes, lifestyle

Type 2 Diabetes Can Be Prevented or Delayed with Lifestyle Changes

According to the Diabetes Prevention Program study:

| modest weight loss (7% of body weight) | + | physical activity (30 minutes per day) | = | 58% reduction in risk for type 2 diabetes |

changes are always the foundation of diabetes prevention.

A key point to remember is that preventing or delaying type 2 diabetes requires only fairly small changes in lifestyle. Notice that success doesn't mean starving yourself to reach an "ideal body weight" or running endless laps. A 7% weight loss translates to losing 14 pounds for someone who weighs 200 pounds. Moderate-intensity physical activity equates to taking a brisk walk for about 30 minutes each day, five days a week.

These goals are small steps toward the bigger reward of good health. As you take these small steps and experience small successes, you will develop more confidence in yourself and your ability to make the changes you need to stay healthy.

Simple Steps for Losing 7% of Your Body Weight

Nutrition goal	Simple step
Lower your calorie intake while maintaining a healthy eating pattern	• Drink water or a sugar-free beverage instead of a regular soda or juice drink. By doing this, you can cut out about 250 calories for each 20-ounce drink. • Choose foods that aren't fried. The calorie and fat savings can be dramatic. A 2 1/2-ounce serving of french fries has almost four times more calories than a baked potato of the same weight because of its fat content.
Eat fewer calories from fat	• Replace high-fat snacks with fruits and vegetables. Keep them cut up and ready to eat on your refrigerator shelf. • Use reduced-fat (light) or fat-free versions of high-fat foods, such as sour cream, cream cheese, mayonnaise, cheese, and salad dressing.
Eat more whole grains and dietary fiber	• Substitute whole-wheat pasta, rice, and bread for the more refined white versions. The fiber will help you feel full, so you will be less likely to overeat. • Go for whole grains such as popcorn, quinoa, and whole oats/oatmeal, which are rich in fiber, vitamins, and minerals.

What Is Moderate-Intensity Physical Activity?

Your heart rate is the number of times your heart beats per minute. Moderate-intensity physical activity causes your heart to beat at 50–70% of your maximum heart rate. According to the American Heart Association, your maximum heart rate is about 220 minus your age. If you're 60 years old, your maximum heart rate is about 160 beats per minute; 50–70% of your maximum heart rate is about 80–112 beats per minute.

Examples of moderate-intensity physical activity include:

- Walking 2 miles in 30 minutes
- Cycling 4 miles in 15 minutes
- Water aerobics for 30 minutes
- Stair walking for 15 minutes
- Gardening for 30–45 minutes
- Raking leaves for 30 minutes

What to Do If You Have Type 2 Diabetes

Type 2 diabetes is a progressive disease. This means that despite your best efforts at lifestyle changes, over time prediabetes can progress to type 2 diabetes, or type 2 diabetes may begin to require treatment with oral medications or injectable medications in addition to healthy eating and physical activity. This doesn't mean you have "bad" diabetes or only had a "mild" case in the beginning. Don't blame yourself if you feel that you didn't take the best possible care of your condition. Would you blame yourself if you needed stronger glasses because your eyesight changed? Because of the progressive nature of diabetes, self-management education with your diabetes team can be customized to provide you with support no matter where you are in your life with diabetes.

When diagnosed with type 2 diabetes, you are at increased risk for many serious complications. Some complications of poorly controlled type 2 diabetes are:

- Heart disease (cardiovascular disease)
- Blindness (retinopathy)

- Nerve damage (neuropathy)
- Kidney damage (nephropathy)

High blood glucose, high blood pressure, and high blood lipids (total cholesterol, LDL cholesterol, and triglycerides) are contributing factors to diabetes complications.

Complications are not always a consequence of high blood glucose. Studies show that the risk for cardiovascular complications is indeed associated with diabetes but is favorably modified by the control of high blood pressure and the treatment of high blood lipids more clearly than by glycemic control. However, glucose control has been shown to have an impact on retinopathy, nephropathy, and neuropathy.

Better health care for those with diabetes has led to the good news that rates of certain diabetes-related complications (heart attacks, ketoacidosis, coma, stroke, amputations, and end-stage kidney disease) have dropped in the past 20 years. The American Diabetes Association has made recommendations for diabetes control based on important clinical research, but remember that these goals need to be personalized for you based on your age, how long you've had diabetes, and your other health conditions (if any).

It's vitally important that you and your diabetes health-care team discuss your personal goals for blood glucose, blood pressure, and blood lipids. Your goals for diabetes control may differ from American Diabetes Association recommendations based on your own individual situation.

American Diabetes Association Recommendations*

Blood Glucose

- Premeal (fasting): 80–130 mg/dL
- 2 hours after meals: <180 mg/dL

A1C (average blood glucose control for the past 2–3 months)

- <7% for most people

Blood Pressure

- <140/90 mmHg for most people

Blood Lipids

- **LDL ("bad") cholesterol:** <100 mg/dL or <70 mg/dL if you already have cardiovascular disease
- **HDL ("good") cholesterol:** >40 mg/dL in men or >50 mg/dL in women
- **Triglycerides:** <150 mg/dL

What Are Your Goals for Diabetes Control?

Discuss your personal goals for diabetes control with your diabetes health-care team and write them here.

Blood glucose	
Premeal (fasting)	
2 hours after meals	
A1C	
Blood pressure	
Blood lipids	
LDL cholesterol	
HDL cholesterol	
Triglycerides	

These goals are provided as a point of reference. Consult with your health-care team to determine whether higher or lower goals are appropriate for you.

Managing Type 2 Diabetes

You won't learn everything you need to know about managing type 2 diabetes just by reading this book or going to one appointment with your diabetes educator. Learning about successful diabetes management is a lifelong process with several areas to master. The American Association of Diabetes Educators (AADE) has developed a list of seven self-care behaviors (see Table 1.1) that you can use to focus your diabetes management. Working with your diabetes educator or diabetes health-care team, you can use these behaviors as a checklist to be certain you've learned about every important area of diabetes self-management.

You can also learn more about managing all aspects of your diabetes by going to the American Diabetes Association's website (at www.diabetes.org) or by reading a good diabetes book, such as *Real-Life Guide to Diabetes, American Diabetes Association Complete Guide to Diabetes,* or *Your First Year with Diabetes, Second Edition* (all available at www.shopdiabetes.org).

Table 1.1	The AADE 7 Self-Care Behaviors
Self-care behavior	**Do you know...**
Healthy eating	the effect of carbohydrate on blood glucose?
	what, when, and how much to eat?
Being active	how often, how long, and at what intensity you should exercise?
	how to balance physical activity with your food and medication?
Monitoring	how often you need to check your blood glucose?
	your target goals for blood glucose, blood pressure, and blood lipids?
Taking medication	the names, doses, and actions of your medications?
	the side effects of your medications?
Problem solving	the symptoms of hyperglycemia (high blood glucose) and hypoglycemia (low blood glucose)?
	how to adjust your food, medication, and physical activity based on your blood glucose levels?
Reducing risks	which tests and exams will enable you to better monitor your health?
	how to prevent the complications of diabetes?
Healthy coping	the benefits of diabetes self-care?
	how to find support for dealing with diabetes?

Behaviors listed are based on those available on the American Association of Diabetes Educators website (www.diabeteseducator.org/ProfessionalResources/AADE7).

Nutrition: A Special Focus in Type 2 Diabetes

Nutrition has long been recognized as the cornerstone for successful diabetes management. Even as far back as 1550 B.C., doctors recommended that people with diabetes follow a diet of wheat grain, fresh grits, grapes, honey berries, and sweet beer to replace the sugar lost through the urine! Today, good nutrition for type 2 diabetes is based on the following nutrition goals and the nutrition recommendations (see Table 1.2) from the American Diabetes Association.

Table 1.2	A Quick Look at the Nutrition Recommendations for Diabetes
Nutrient or food source	**Nutrition recommendation for diabetes**
Calories	You may need to reduce the number of calories you eat to lower your blood glucose and promote weight loss. Removing just 500 calories from your daily intake could mean a weight loss of one pound each week.
Carbohydrate	The amount (grams) of carbohydrate and available insulin have a strong influence on the way your blood glucose reacts after you eat. Monitoring your total grams of carbohydrate, by using either food choices, carbohydrate counting, or estimates, is a key strategy to improve your blood glucose control. See Chapter 2 for more details.
Fiber and Whole Grains	Your fiber and whole grain goals should be the same amount recommended for the other members of your family: about 25 grams of fiber per day for adult women and 38 grams of fiber per day for adult men. At least half of all the grains you eat should be whole grains. See Chapter 8 for more details.
Protein	If you have normal kidney function, your intake of protein foods (meats, poultry, seafood, dairy foods, beans, peas, nuts, and seeds) should be the same as that of the general public. See Chapter 8 for more details.
Fat	There is no proven ideal *quantity* of fat recommended for those with diabetes; however, *quality* or type of fat is important to maintain heart health. Foods higher in unsaturated fats (liquid fats) are better for you than saturated and trans fats. See Chapter 8 for more details. A nutrition professional can help you learn more about heart-healthy unsaturated fats and how to avoid saturated and trans fats, as well as identify the right amount of fat for you. Modifying the quality and quantity of your fat intake may help lower your risk for heart attack and stroke. Lower fat intake can also translate into lower calorie intake, which may help you maintain a reasonable body weight.
Vitamins, Minerals, and Herbal Supplements	The American Diabetes Association does not recommend any special vitamins, minerals, or herbal supplements for most individuals with diabetes.

(continued on next page)

Table 1.2	A Quick Look at the Nutrition Recommendations for Diabetes *(Continued)*
Alcohol	If you choose to drink alcohol, use it in moderation: one drink or fewer per day if you're a woman or two drinks or fewer per day if you're a man. Alcohol may increase your risk for hypoglycemia. See Chapter 10 for more details.
Sodium	Sodium recommendations for people with diabetes are similar to those for the general population: <2,300 milligrams per day. See Chapter 8 for more details.
Sweeteners	A number of zero-calorie and reduced-calorie sweeteners are approved for use in the U.S. People with diabetes are advised to limit or avoid sugar-sweetened beverages to reduce the risk of weight gain and cardiovascular disease. See Chapter 2 and Chapter 9 for more details.

Although this quick overview of nutrition recommendations for diabetes can help you get started, it's best to meet with a nutrition professional to develop an individualized meal plan based on your needs, goals, and personal food preferences.

Evert et al. Nutrition therapy recommendations for the management of adults with diabetes. *Diabetes Care* 2014;37(Suppl. 1):S120–143.

American Diabetes Association Nutrition Goals

- Attain individualized blood glucose, blood pressure, and lipid goals. General recommended goals from the American Diabetes Association are as follows:
  - A1C <7%
  - Blood pressure <140/90 mmHg
  - Blood lipids:
    - LDL cholesterol <100 mg/dL
    - Triglycerides <150 mg/dL
    - HDL cholesterol >40 mg/dL for men
    - HDL cholesterol >50 mg/dL for women
- Achieve and maintain body weight goals.
- Delay or prevent complications of diabetes.
- Address individual nutrition needs.
- Maintain the pleasure of eating.
- Learn about practical tools for day-to-day meal planning rather than focusing on individual nutrients or single foods.

Weighty Issues

The vast majority of individuals with type 2 diabetes are overweight and have insulin resistance. They also often have high blood pressure and high blood lipids. Weight loss is an important part of therapy for improving all aspects of

Partners in Health: Your Registered Dietitian/Registered Dietitian Nutritionist and Certified Diabetes Educator

The American Diabetes Association's nutrition goals provide you with very general guidelines. You will find step-by-step advice on the important details of reaching these goals as you delve further into *What Do I Eat Now?* But the best place to find the individualized and personalized advice you need to ensure healthy eating success is by working with your registered dietitian (RD)/registered dietitian nutritionist (RDN) and/or certified diabetes educator (CDE).

An RD/RDN may provide additional advice on how to incorporate physical activity into your life as well. For a referral to an RD/RDN, ask your physician or locate one near you through the Academy of Nutrition and Dietetics website (www.eatright.org). Many RD/RDN's are also certified diabetes educators, and they can help you understand how any diabetes medications you're taking affect you, can teach you how to monitor your blood glucose, and can teach you how to solve problems and adjust emotionally to diabetes. You can ask your physician for referral to a CDE or locate one through the American Association of Diabetes Educators website (www.diabeteseducator.org) or by entering your zip code under "Find a CDE" on the National Certification Board for Diabetes Educators website (www.ncbde.org).

How often should you see these important partners in health? If you're newly diagnosed with type 2 diabetes, three or four visits can get your diabetes meal plan off to a great start. After that, a visit every year should help you stay on track and keep you up-to-date on the latest developments in the area of healthy eating for diabetes.

Spending a bit of time and money on visits with an RD/RDN or CDE is a great investment in your future. Because nutrition is a key factor in helping to control your diabetes, eating healthfully will improve blood glucose now and may help prevent costly complications and expensive medical care later in life!

type 2 diabetes. Just as in the treatment of pre-diabetes, small changes can yield big results.

If your weight is a concern, you can start managing it by determining your weight status. A measurement known as the body mass index (BMI) takes into account your height and weight, making it a reliable indicator of body fat. **You can find your BMI by using:**

- An online BMI calculator. You can find an excellent BMI calculator at the website for the National Heart, Lung, and

Table 1.3   Body Mass Index

BMI	Normal						Overweight					Obese					
	19	20	21	22	23	24	25	26	27	28	29	30	31	32	33	34	35
Height (inches)	Body weight (pounds)																
58	91	96	100	105	110	115	119	124	129	134	138	143	148	153	158	162	167
59	94	99	104	109	114	119	124	128	133	138	143	148	153	158	163	168	173
60	97	102	107	112	118	123	128	133	138	143	148	153	158	163	168	174	179
61	100	106	111	116	122	127	132	137	143	148	153	158	164	169	174	180	185
62	104	109	115	120	126	131	136	142	147	153	158	164	169	175	180	186	191
63	107	113	118	124	130	135	141	146	152	158	163	169	175	180	186	191	197
64	110	116	122	128	134	140	145	151	157	163	169	174	180	186	192	197	204
65	114	120	126	132	138	144	150	156	162	168	174	180	186	192	198	204	210
66	118	124	130	136	142	148	155	161	167	173	179	186	192	198	204	210	216
67	121	127	134	140	146	153	159	166	172	178	185	191	198	204	211	217	223
68	125	131	138	144	151	158	164	171	177	184	190	197	203	210	216	223	230
69	128	135	142	149	155	162	169	176	182	189	196	203	209	216	223	230	236
70	132	139	146	153	160	167	174	181	188	195	202	209	216	222	229	236	243
71	136	143	150	157	165	172	179	186	193	200	208	215	222	229	236	243	250
72	140	147	154	162	169	177	184	191	199	206	213	221	228	235	242	250	258
73	144	151	159	166	174	182	189	197	204	212	219	227	235	242	250	257	265
74	148	155	163	171	179	186	194	202	210	218	225	233	241	249	256	264	272
75	152	160	168	176	184	192	200	208	216	224	232	240	248	256	264	272	279
76	156	164	172	180	189	197	205	213	221	230	238	246	254	263	271	279	287

National Institutes of Health. Body mass index table. Available from http://www.nhlbi.nih.gov/health/educational/lose_wt/BMI/bmi_tbl.pdf.

Blood Institute (www.nhlbi.nih.gov/guidelines/obesity/BMI/bmicalc.htm).

- An adult BMI chart (see Table 1.3). Locate your height in the left column and read across the row for that height to find your weight. Follow the column of the weight up to the top row that lists your BMI.
- Calculate it yourself. Multiply your weight in pounds by 703 and then divide by your height in inches squared. The formula looks like this:

$$\frac{weight\,(pounds) \times 703}{[height\,(inches) \times height\,(inches)]}$$

For example, if you're 5′5″ (65 inches) tall and weigh 180 pounds, here's how you'd calculate your BMI:

$$\frac{180 \times 703}{[65 \times 65]} = About\ 30\ BMI$$

				Extreme obesity														
36	37	38	39	40	41	42	43	44	45	46	47	48	49	50	51	52	53	54
172	177	181	186	191	196	201	205	210	215	220	224	229	234	239	244	248	253	258
178	183	188	193	198	203	208	212	217	222	227	232	237	242	247	252	257	262	267
184	189	194	199	204	209	215	220	225	230	235	240	245	250	255	261	266	271	276
190	195	201	206	211	217	222	227	232	238	243	248	254	259	264	269	275	280	285
196	202	207	213	218	224	229	235	240	246	251	256	262	267	273	278	284	289	295
203	208	214	220	225	231	237	242	248	254	259	265	270	278	282	287	293	299	304
209	215	221	227	232	238	244	250	256	262	267	273	279	285	291	296	302	308	314
216	222	228	234	240	246	252	258	264	270	276	282	288	294	300	306	312	318	324
223	229	235	241	247	253	260	266	272	278	284	291	297	303	309	315	322	328	334
230	236	242	249	255	261	268	274	280	287	293	299	306	312	319	325	331	338	344
236	243	249	256	262	269	276	282	289	295	302	308	315	322	328	335	341	348	354
243	250	257	263	270	277	284	291	297	304	311	318	324	331	338	345	351	358	365
250	257	264	271	278	285	292	299	306	313	320	327	334	341	348	355	362	369	376
257	265	272	279	286	293	301	308	315	322	329	338	343	351	358	365	372	379	386
265	272	279	287	294	302	309	316	324	331	338	346	353	361	368	375	383	390	397
272	280	288	295	302	310	318	325	333	340	348	355	363	371	378	386	393	401	408
280	287	295	303	311	319	326	334	342	350	358	365	373	381	389	396	404	412	420
287	295	303	311	319	327	335	343	351	359	367	375	383	391	399	407	415	423	431
295	304	312	320	328	336	344	353	361	369	377	385	394	402	410	418	426	435	443

Use your BMI to pinpoint your weight status and potential health concerns.

BMI	Weight status
<18.5	Underweight
18.5–24.9	Normal weight
25.0–29.9	Overweight*
≥30	Obese

Recent findings note that Asian Americans are at an increased risk for diabetes at lower BMI levels relative to the general population. "Overweight" for Asian Americans is a BMI of 23 vs. 25.

As body fat or BMI increases, health risks increase. Being overweight (BMI of 25–29.9) or being obese (BMI ≥30) increases the risk of having high blood pressure, heart disease, stroke, diabetes, certain types of cancer, arthritis, and breathing problems. Research shows that being obese lowers your life expectancy.

Which Meal Plan Is Best for Diabetes and Weight Loss?

There are many, many approaches to losing weight. In fact, if you do a Google search of "how to lose weight," over 100 million entries appear! Which weight-loss approach is best for people with diabetes? Certainly, losing those extra pounds is an important first step to managing type 2 diabetes, and the best approach to use for weight loss is the one that enables you to keep the weight off forever.

Diabetes nutrition recommendations are now focusing more on healthful eating patterns (combinations of different nutrient-dense foods and food groups including starch, fruits, milk and milk substitutes, nonstarchy vegetables, protein, fats, sweets/desserts, and other carbohydrates) than on single nutrients such as carbohydrate, fat, or sodium. A variety of eating patterns are acceptable for the manage-

ment of diabetes, and your personal preferences and diabetes goals are important considerations when choosing an eating pattern to follow. Table 1.4 describes some of the most common eating patterns and provides a few sample food ideas.

While more research is needed, each of these eating patterns has shown varying levels of success in improving glucose control and cardiovascular risk factors and helping with weight loss—particularly if calories, carbohydrate, and portion sizes are monitored. Work with your nutrition professional to determine which eating pattern is the best for you based on your personal preferences and diabetes goals.

Table 1.4	Eating Patterns for Diabetes and Weight Loss	
Eating pattern	**Description**	**Menu ideas**
Mediterranean	Mediterranean-style eating patterns include lots of plant-based foods (fruits, vegetables, breads, cereals, beans, nuts, and seeds); minimally processed, seasonally fresh, and locally grown foods; fresh fruits as the typical daily dessert; sugar or honey eaten only on special occasions; olive oil as the principal source of fat; dairy products (mainly cheese and yogurt) eaten in low to moderate amounts; fewer than 4 eggs per week; red meat eaten infrequently and in small amounts; and wine in low to moderate amounts, generally with meals.	Breakfast: Greek yogurt topped with berries and walnuts, cubed cantaloupe

Lunch: White bean soup, hummus and vegetables in a whole-wheat pita

Dinner: Grilled salmon stuffed with spinach and feta cheese, wheat berry salad (olive oil, vinaigrette, feta, parsley, and tomatoes), baked apples with cherries and almonds, glass of red wine (if you choose to drink wine)

Snacks: Nuts, whole-grain crackers and cheese |

(continued on next page)

Table 1.4	Eating Patterns for Diabetes and Weight Loss *(Continued)*	
Eating pattern	**Description**	**Menu ideas**
Vegetarian and Vegan	Vegan meal plans don't contain any flesh foods or animal-derived products; vegetarian meal plans don't include flesh foods but may include eggs (ovo) and/or dairy (lacto) products. These eating patterns feature lower intakes of saturated fat and cholesterol and higher intakes of fruits, vegetables, whole grains, nuts, soy products, fiber, and phytochemicals.	***Vegan Meals*** Breakfast: Whole-grain cereal with soy milk, banana Lunch: Grilled vegetable sandwich (tomatoes, zucchini, peppers, onion, garlic, and beans), green spinach salad with vinaigrette dressing Dinner: Tofu stir-fry with sautéed vegetables (such as broccoli, snow peas, baby corn, water chestnuts), soy yogurt parfait Snacks: Fresh fruits and vegetables, soy or almond milk fruit smoothie ***Vegetarian Meals*** Variations on the vegan meals above that may include eggs and dairy products
Low Fat	Low-fat meal plans emphasize vegetables, fruits, starches (breads/crackers, pasta, whole grains, starchy vegetables), lean protein, and low-fat dairy products. In this eating pattern, total fat intake is <30% of calories and saturated fat intake is <10% of calories.	Breakfast: Whole-grain english muffin with fat-free cream cheese, blueberries, skim milk Lunch: Chicken noodle soup, green salad with chicken and fat-free french dressing, fresh pineapple Dinner: Grilled shrimp skewers on brown rice, tossed salad with fat-free caesar dressing, watermelon Snacks: Fat-free yogurt, low-fat cheese with whole-wheat crackers

(continued on next page)

Table 1.4	Eating Patterns for Diabetes and Weight Loss *(Continued)*	
Eating pattern	**Description**	**Menu ideas**
Low Carbohydrate	Low-carbohydrate meal plans focus on foods higher in protein (meat, poultry, fish, shellfish, eggs, cheese, nuts, seeds), fats (oils, butter, olives, avocado), and vegetables that are low in carbohydrate (salad greens, cucumbers, broccoli, summer squash). Most plans allow fruit and higher-carbohydrate vegetables; however, added sugar–containing foods and grain products (such as pasta, rice, couscous, tortillas, and breads) are generally avoided. The amount of carbohydrate allowed varies depending on the specific plan and the individual's needs. There doesn't seem to be a consistent definition of "low carbohydrate," but the amount of carbohydrate eaten may range from very low (21–70 g/day of carbohydrate) to moderately low (30–40% of calories from carbohydrates).	Breakfast: Eggs cooked in canola oil, canadian bacon, fresh grapefruit Lunch: Sliced grilled chicken wrapped in lettuce with tomatoes and mayonnaise, romaine lettuce salad with avocado slices and vinaigrette dressing Dinner: London broil, mushrooms sautéed in oil, spinach salad with pecans and blue cheese dressing, sugar-free gelatin Snack: Whole almonds, string cheese
DASH (Dietary Approaches to Stop Hypertension)	The DASH eating pattern emphasizes fruits, vegetables, and low-fat dairy products, including whole grains, poultry, fish, and nuts. It limits saturated fat, red meat, sweets, and sugar-containing beverages. The most effective DASH meal plan is also low in sodium.	Breakfast: Cooked oatmeal with low-fat milk, low-sodium vegetable juice, banana Lunch: Unsalted chicken salad on whole-wheat bread with dijon mustard, apple, low-fat milk Dinner: Baked turkey, broccoli, whole-wheat roll with unsalted soft margarine, fat-free yogurt Snacks: Unsalted almonds or pretzels, fresh fruits and vegetables

Adapted from Evert et al. Nutrition therapy recommendations for the management of adults with diabetes. *Diabetes Care* 2014;37(Suppl. 1):S120–143.

Create Your Plate

Another helpful meal planning tool for those recently diagnosed with diabetes is called "Create Your Plate." This tool is an easy way for people with diabetes to control portion sizes and limit their intake of starchy foods.

Follow these seven easy steps to Create Your Plate:

1. Using your dinner plate, put a line down the middle of the plate. Then on one side, cut it again so you will have three sections on your plate.

2. Fill the largest section with colorful non-starchy vegetables such as:
   - Spinach, carrots, lettuce, greens, cabbage, bok choy
   - Green beans, broccoli, cauliflower, tomatoes
   - Vegetable juice, salsa, onion, cucumber, beets, okra
   - Mushrooms, peppers, turnips

3. Now in one of the small sections, put grains and starchy foods such as:
   - Whole-grain breads, such as whole wheat or rye
   - Whole-grain, high-fiber cereal
   - Cooked cereal such as oatmeal, grits, hominy, or cream of wheat
   - Rice, pasta, dal, tortillas
   - Cooked starchy beans and peas, such as pinto beans or black-eyed peas
   - Potatoes, green peas, corn, lima beans, sweet potatoes, winter squash
   - Low-fat crackers, snack chips, pretzels, and light popcorn

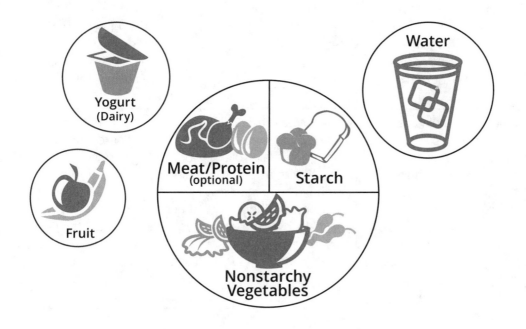

4. And then in the other small section, put your protein-rich foods such as:
    o Chicken or turkey without the skin
    o Fish such as tuna, salmon, cod, or catfish
    o Other seafood such as shrimp, clams, oysters, crab, or mussels
    o Lean cuts of beef and pork such as sirloin or pork loin
    o Tofu, eggs, low-fat cheese
5. Add a serving of fruit, a serving of dairy, or both as your meal plan allows.
6. Choose healthy fats in small amounts. For cooking, use oils. For salads, some healthy additions are nuts, seeds, avocado, and vinaigrettes.
7. To complete your meal, add a low-calorie drink like water, unsweetened tea, or coffee.

Lifestyle Changes That Work for Weight Loss!

No matter which eating pattern or weight-loss options you choose, lifestyle changes based on healthy eating, physical activity, and behavior change are the foundation of any successful weight-loss program. **Here are a few examples of lifestyle changes you can make to promote weight loss:**

Healthy eating	Physical activity	Behavior change
Monitor your weight and blood glucose every day. It's much easier to make small, daily corrections to your food and activity level than to try to offset a larger weight gain or elevated A1C.	Walk at least 10,000 steps a day; use a pedometer or activity tracker to count your steps.	Nothing motivates like success! Setting concrete and achievable goals, such as eating fruit at breakfast or replacing an after-dinner TV show with a walk, can build up your confidence to change your behavior for the better.
Lower your fat intake to lower your calories. For example, using skim milk instead of whole milk saves 56 calories per cup, which translates into almost 18 pounds of weight lost over a year, if you drink three glasses a day.	Look for ways to increase your heart rate during your daily routine. Walk to a nearby errand instead of taking a car or bus. Choose the stairs over the escalator or elevator.	Change your eating style to make it easier to eat less without feeling deprived. It takes 20 or more minutes for your brain to get the message that you've been fed. Eating slowly will help you feel satisfied. Changing your eating schedule, or setting one, can be helpful, especially if you tend to skip or delay meals and overeat later.

Healthy eating	Physical activity	Behavior change
Eat the rainbow! Make half of your plate nonstarchy vegetables. Include a variety of colorful fruits and vegetables, which are packed with fiber, vitamins, and minerals. (See examples in "Create Your Plate" on page 17.)	If you don't have time to exercise the recommended 30 minutes per day all at one time, break up your physical activity to three 10-minute sessions each day. You'll still reap the benefits of the activity.	Keep your workout clothes and shoes in the car so you're always prepared when an opportunity to exercise presents itself.

Other Options?

In addition to healthy eating, physical activity, and behavior change, other options for weight loss include:

- *Weight-loss medications,* which can help you achieve a loss of 5–10% of weight when combined with lifestyle changes. Some of these medications have unpleasant side effects, and, of course, they only work when you take them. Medications are generally only recommended for those with a BMI >27 (other weight-related factors may be taken into consideration in addition to BMI).
- *Bariatric surgery* may be a consideration if your BMI is >35 and your diabetes or associated comorbidites are difficult to control with lifestyle changes and medication. Although bariatric surgery has been shown to lead to near or complete normalization of blood glucose in about

40–95% of patients with type 2 diabetes, it is a costly and potentially risky approach to weight loss. It's not regarded as a "cure" for type 2 diabetes, so those who have had a bariatric procedure need lifelong lifestyle support and medical monitoring, including regular screenings of their blood glucose.

Putting It All Together

Many people with diabetes aren't able to see a registered dietitian/registered dietitian nutritionist or certified diabetes educator immediately after being diagnosed with diabetes. But if that's your situation, you can still get started on the path to balanced eating and learn more about the basics of good nutrition before you attend your first appointment with a nutrition professional.

Take advantage of a great online nutrition resource from the American Diabetes Association—the "Food & Fitness" page on the Association's website (available at www. diabetes.org/food-and-fitness). The American Diabetes Association site is brimming with food tips, meal planning tools, shopping lists, and recipes, as well as a guide to healthy eating and physical activity that can lead to better blood glucose control. Another important feature included on the site is "Create Your Plate" (previously reviewed on page 17).

The United States Department of Agriculture (USDA) also has a wealth of no-cost information about healthy eating for the general public as well as meal plans for weight loss on the Choose My Plate website (available at www.choosemyplate.gov). While not diabetes-specific, this online resource includes a step-by-step approach to weight management, which includes tips on determining your current eating habits, an online SuperTracker, guidance on what to eat and drink along with personalized Daily Food Plans, and tips for making better food choices while at home or eating out. Check out the "Weight and Calories" page of the website to access these features.

It Starts with a Single Step

Small steps lead to big achievements. Whether your nutrition goal is to lose weight or lower your blood glucose, it won't happen on its own. First, think about each action you need to take to achieve your goal; then, divide it into small steps that are easy to achieve. After you complete several small steps, you will have achieved your overall goal. For example, if your goal is to eat less fast food and cook more meals at home, you should:

- Set aside time to make healthful eating a priority.
- Plan menus and choose recipes.
- Shop so you have the ingredients in your kitchen to prepare healthy recipes.
- Rediscover the lost art of cooking to minimize the use of prepackaged foods.

It's been said that whoever wants to reach a distant goal must take small steps. Let's move forward and take the next steps!

Next Steps

Review the nutrition goals you set in the Introduction. Choose your highest-priority nutrition goal and list three changes you can make today to help you move toward accomplishing that goal.

My highest-priority nutrition goal is:

_____

_____

_____

The three steps I will take TODAY to reach that goal are:

1. _____
_____

2. _____
_____

3. _____
_____

What Do I Eat for Dinner?

FOR 45–60 GRAMS OF CARBOHYDRATE*

Recipe: Salmon and Asparagus Foil Packet
(1 serving)

1/2 cup wild rice

3/4 cup citrus fruit salad (white/red grapefruit
and orange sections)

FOR 60–75 GRAMS OF CARBOHYDRATE*

Recipe: Salmon and Asparagus Foil Packet
(1 serving)

1/2 cup wild rice

1 slice sourdough bread

3/4 cup citrus fruit salad (white/red grapefruit
and orange sections)

*For most women, 45–60 grams of carbohydrate at a meal is a good starting point; for most men, 60–75 grams of carbohydrate per meal is appropriate. Check with your diabetes health-care team to find the amount of carbohydrate that's right for you.

Swift, Simple Tips

- You can buy sourdough bread (in rolls or loaves of various shapes and sizes) in the bakery or health food section of most grocery stores. It's traditionally a white bread, but whole-wheat and rye versions are available. Choose the whole-grain variety whenever possible.
- No time to prepare a citrus fruit salad? Check out your grocer's produce section for chilled, ready-to-serve mixtures of white/red grapefruit and orange sections.

SALMON AND ASPARAGUS FOIL PACKETS

SERVES: 4

SERVING SIZE: 1 packet

PREPARATION TIME: 20–25 minutes

COOKING TIME: 15–18 minutes

INGREDIENTS

1 pound fresh asparagus

4 sheets 12 × 18-inch heavy-duty foil wrap

Nonstick cooking spray

4 (5-ounce) fillets skinless salmon

2 tablespoons low-sodium soy sauce

2 teaspoons freshly squeezed lemon juice

2 tablespoons packed light brown sugar

1 tablespoon honey

1 teaspoon bottled minced fresh garlic

1 teaspoon sesame seeds

1. Preheat oven to 450°F.
2. Break ends off asparagus spears and divide spears into four portions.
3. Spray center of each foil sheet with nonstick cooking spray. Place one salmon fillet in the middle of each sheet of foil along with 1/4 of the asparagus.
4. Combine low-sodium soy sauce, lemon juice, brown sugar, honey, and garlic in a small bowl. Drizzle 1/4 of mixture on top of salmon and asparagus in each foil packet. Sprinkle 1/4 teaspoon of sesame seeds on top of salmon and asparagus in each packet.
5. Bring up sides of foil and fold the top over twice. Seal the ends, leaving room for air to circulate inside the packet. Place packets on a cookie sheet and bake for 15–18 minutes, until salmon is opaque. Be careful opening packets; moisture creates steam during cooking, which can burn your hand if you quickly tear open the foil.

Recipe Tip

- Don't want to heat up the kitchen? Foil packets are great for grilling! Grill over medium-low heat. Cover grill and cook 13–16 minutes, rotating packets 1/2 turn after about 7 minutes. Have a baking sheet or large plate handy to hold your packets once they're done cooking.

CHOICES/EXCHANGES	BASIC NUTRITIONAL VALUES			
1 Carbohydrate,	**Calories**	280	**Potassium**	700 mg
5 Lean Protein	Calories from Fat	80	**Total Carbohydrate**	15 g
	Total Fat	9.0 g	Dietary Fiber	2 g
	Saturated Fat	1.9 g	Sugars	12 g
	Trans Fat	0.0 g	**Protein**	33 g
	Cholesterol	65 mg	**Phosphorus**	385 mg
	Sodium	350 mg		

Food for Thought

- **Type 2 diabetes is a progressive condition.** Healthy eating, physical activity, and behavior changes are the foundation for diabetes treatment, but new therapies and medications may need to be added to your diabetes-care plan over time.
- **Type 2 diabetes responds well to weight loss, healthy eating, and physical activity.**
- **The healthy eating guidelines for people with type 2 diabetes are the same as those for everyone in your family:**
  - Eat high-fiber grains, beans, fruits, and vegetables.
  - Consume small portions of meat and protein foods.
  - Limit your intake of fats, refined starches, sweets, and alcohol.

H ave you heard any of this advice from well-intentioned family members, friends, or acquaintances?

"You can't eat sugar or sweets anymore."
*"Avoid bananas and oranges because they'll make your blood glucose
    levels too high."*
"No more potatoes or carrots for you."
"Skip the bread and pasta."

The good news is that *none of these recommendations are actually true* when it comes to healthy eating with diabetes. Granted, the foods mentioned above are rich in carbohydrate, and, as you may know, carbohydrate raises blood glucose levels. But carbohydrate-containing foods do *not* have to be totally avoided when you have diabetes.

Why the Concern about Carbohydrate?

So, what is the story on carbohydrate? Most people with diabetes enjoy carbohydrate foods—a plate of pasta, warm crusty rolls, gooey chocolate brownies, a tall glass of cold milk, a colorful bowl of berries, or fresh-squeezed orange juice. But figuring out how much carbohydrate and which carbohydrate foods to eat are important decisions you'll need to make every day. Before you can really know what or how much to eat, a basic understanding of what carbohydrate is and its impact on diabetes is just what the diabetes educator ordered.

Carbohydrate is one of three key energy-containing nutrients—or building blocks—that make up all of the foods you eat. The other two building blocks are protein and fat. (You'll learn more about protein and fat in Chapter 8.) Your body needs all three nutrients to be healthy. Keep in mind that because each of these three provides fuel for your body, they can contribute to weight gain. And, as discussed in Chapter 1, weight gain can contribute to insulin resistance and the worsening of average overall glucose control.

While carbohydrate, protein, and fat all provide fuel for your body, carbohydrate is your body's preferred fuel. Carbohydrate gets the most attention when it comes to diabetes because carbohydrate is the component of your meals and snacks that is most directly responsible for the rise in blood glucose after eating. Protein and fat do not affect your after-meal blood glucose rise to anywhere near the same extent as carbohydrate does.

As you read on, you'll learn more about which foods and beverages contain carbohydrate, and how much carbohydrate they contain. You'll also learn some general basics about how to control your carbohydrate intake each day.

Carbohydrate at Work In Your Body

Simply put, when you eat foods or drink beverages that contain carbohydrate, your body breaks that carbohydrate down into glucose (a type of sugar), which then raises the level of glucose in your blood in order to fuel your body. Eating too much carbohydrate may raise your blood glucose too high. *But* too little carbohydrate may cause your blood glucose to drop too low, especially if you take diabetes medicines that lower blood glucose.

Carbohydrate begins to raise blood glucose levels within 15–20 minutes of eating. Maybe you've already noticed that you feel "different" a few minutes after you eat—that may be due to your blood glucose level rising. Before you had diabetes, after eating a meal or snack, your body could sense the glucose

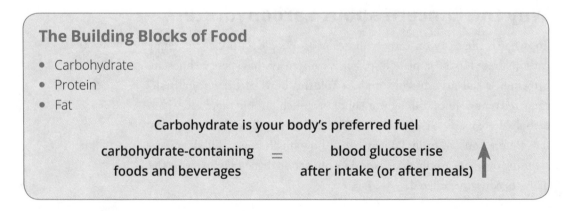

The Building Blocks of Food

- Carbohydrate
- Protein
- Fat

Carbohydrate is your body's preferred fuel

carbohydrate-containing foods and beverages = **blood glucose rise after intake (or after meals)**

coming from the carbohydrate you ate and would automatically regulate the amount of glucose in your bloodstream. Now that you have type 2 diabetes, your body is no longer able to automatically keep the right amount of glucose in your bloodstream, so the more carbohydrate you eat, the higher your blood glucose level may rise (unless you take action to change it). Blood glucose levels peak about 1 1/2–2 hours after you begin eating. Then they should begin to drop. Controlling your carbohydrate intake helps reduce that after-meal blood glucose peak, with the goal of keeping your blood glucose in your target range.

Blood Glucose Targets

In general, the American Diabetes Association recommendations for blood glucose targets are as follows:

- Before a meal: 80–130 mg/dL
- 1–2 hours after the start of the meal: <180 mg/dL

Make sure you consult with your diabetes health-care team to determine what blood glucose targets are safest for you.

Just because carbohydrate raises blood glucose doesn't mean you should eliminate carbohydrate from your diet. Your body requires carbohydrate each day to stay strong and healthy. Studies examining the ideal amount of carbohydrate intake for people with diabetes are inconclusive. With that said, drastically limiting your carbohydrate intake may leave you feeling weak and lethargic. (Remember, carbohydrate is your body's preferred fuel.) Many carbohydrate-containing foods are healthy foods. They not only taste good and fuel your body, but also provide important vitamins, minerals, and fiber that your body needs.

Blood Glucose Control Is a Balancing Act

There are three key components to blood glucose control:

1. Carbohydrate intake: raises blood glucose
2. Diabetes medications: lower blood glucose
3. Physical activity: lowers blood glucose (whether it's walking, working out at the gym, playing sports, gardening, or cleaning the house)

To keep your blood glucose from going too high or too low, you need to balance:

- The amount of carbohydrate you eat
- The amount, types, and timing of the diabetes medicines you take (consult with your diabetes health-care team)
- The amount, type, and timing of physical activity you do

Keeping It Real: Real-Life Situation

It is sometimes difficult to keep your carbohydrate intake, diabetes medications (if any), and physical activity in balance. If you're going to be doing physical activity—such as spending the afternoon doing heavy gardening or yard work, or working out at the gym—you may need extra carbohydrate to maintain your blood glucose level, especially if you take diabetes medications that may cause hypoglycemia (low blood glucose). Ask your pharmacist about any diabetes medication(s) you take if you are unsure whether they may put you at risk for hypoglycemia. Check your blood glucose frequently before, during, and after activity and any time that you experience symptoms of hypoglycemia. Make sure you are familiar with the symptoms of hypoglycemia (see below), and always treat hypoglycemia immediately.

Hypoglycemia is defined as blood glucose <70 mg/dL. If you have hypoglycemia, the following steps can help you stabilize your blood glucose:

- Treat with 15 grams of carbohydrate
- Wait 15 minutes then re-check your blood glucose

- If blood glucose is still under 70 mg/dL, treat with another 15 grams of carbohydrate

Symptoms of hypoglycemia include:

- Shakiness
- Nervousness or anxiety
- Sweating
- Clamminess
- Irritability or impatience
- Confusion
- Rapid/fast heartbeat
- Lightheadedness or dizziness
- Hunger and nausea
- Sleepiness
- Blurred/impaired vision
- Tingling or numbness in the lips or tongue
- Headaches
- Weakness or fatigue
- Anger, stubbornness, or sadness
- Lack of coordination

Talk with your diabetes health-care team about a plan to manage your carbohydrate intake and any diabetes medications to keep your blood glucose in balance during physical activity.

Carbohydrate Control, Consistency, and Counting!

Whether you eat at home or dine out, counting and controlling the carbohydrate you eat and drink is a key strategy to help you control your blood glucose (especially your after-meal blood glucose), feel well, and manage your diabetes.

Carbohydrate Control

The period right after you are diagnosed with type 2 diabetes can be an overwhelming time as you try to sift through and process tons of new information. When it comes to eating, the good news (as you learned in Chapter 1) is that there's no one "diet" or ideal amount of carbohydrate (or protein and fat, for that matter) that everyone with diabetes should eat, just as there's no one perfect diet for people without diabetes. With that said, *carbohydrate control is a priority.* The amount of carbohydrate best suited to you to keep your blood glucose in target should factor in your current eating patterns, preferences, and health goals. For instance, if you're a runner or work in a physically active job, you may need more carbohydrate and at different times of day than if you're trying to drop a few pounds and tend to be physically inactive.

Carbohydrate Consistency

Another key thing to remember: The more consistent your carbohydrate intake is from meal to meal and day to day, the more stable your blood glucose levels are likely to be, particularly your after-meal blood glucose. And in the end, that translates into better diabetes control.

Carbohydrate Counting

To control carbohydrate and maintain consistency, you can track the grams of carbohydrate consumed at each meal and snack (whether from food or beverages). This approach to tracking carbohydrate and maintaining carbohydrate consistency from meal to meal, day to day, is rightfully called "carbohydrate counting." Greater explanation of carbohydrate counting will follow later in this chapter.

While this book focuses primarily on tracking or measuring carbohydrate in grams (abbreviated as g), you may also run across—and can use, if you wish—a unit of measure known as a carbohydrate choice (or serving). Here are some simple tips to help you understand these two different carbohydrate measurements:

- One carbohydrate choice (or serving) = 15 grams of carbohydrate
- To arrive at the number of carbohydrate choices (servings) in a food, take the grams of carbohydrate and divide by 15.
- Alternatively, to get the number of carbohydrate grams from the carbohydrate choices (servings), take the number of carbohydrate choices and multiply by 15.

Over the years, we've had many patients come to us and say they eat three or four "carbs"

> ## Carbohydrate Considerations If You Take Insulin (Injection or Pump)
>
> **If you're on insulin and take a set dose(s) each meal/day,** it's especially important to eat a similar amount of carbohydrate at consistent times each day to coordinate with insulin doses. Skipping meals (or skipping planned snacks) may actually increase your risk for hypoglycemia (low blood glucose).
>
> **If you take multiple daily injections of insulin or use an insulin pump,** you have more flexibility in timing of meals and carbohydrate intake because you can control when and how much you eat and how much insulin you take based on your carbohydrate intake.

at a meal. We've learned that they actually mean three or four carbohydrate choices, not grams of carbohydrate. It's easy to get confused.

3 Steps to Carbohydrate Control

Now let's take a look at three important steps to carbohydrate control. You'll also find specific guidelines and tips in this section to get you started with carbohydrate control no matter which eating pattern or meal plan you choose to follow (see "Eating Patterns for Diabetes and Weight Loss" in Chapter 1). Whether you choose to monitor your carbohydrate intake through carbohydrate counting or simply by estimation based on experience, these steps and tips can help. Your diabetes health-care team can provide further guidance about what's best for you.

Step 1: Get Familiar with Which Foods and Beverages Contain Carbohydrate

First things first. You have to know which foods and beverages contain carbohydrate before you can work on consistency with your carbohydrate intake. Carbohydrate is found in many of the foods we eat. While some foods, like honey, are pure carbohydrate, many foods contain a combination of carbohydrate, protein, and/or fat. For instance, peanut butter is a mix of all three nutrients, and chicken is primarily protein with a little fat. However, as you can see in "Where Can You Find Carbohydrate?" on the next page, many foods contain at least some carbohydrate.

For good health, try to include a variety of carbohydrate-containing foods at meals and snacks each day. If you have a sweet tooth, the really good news is that you can even work

Where Can You Find Carbohydrate?

- Breads and tortillas
- Crackers, chips, and pretzels
- Cereals
- Rice and grains
- Pasta
- Beans, lentils, and plant-based proteins (such as soy-based foods)
- Starchy vegetables (such as sweet and white potatoes, corn, peas, winter squash)
- Fruits and fruit juices
- Yogurt, milk, and milk substitutes (such as soy milk or rice drink)
- Nonstarchy vegetables (such as broccoli, carrots, salad greens, and tomatoes)
- Sweets and desserts (many sugar-free desserts still contain carbohydrate)
- Other combination foods (such as soups and casseroles)

sweets into your meal plan. Sugar is not the evil that it was once thought to be for people with diabetes. Now you truly can have your cake and eat it too—at least in small amounts (see "Are Sweet Treats Off Limits?" on the next page)!

Carbohydrate in Food Groups

Since the total amount of carbohydrate eaten is the primary predictor of after-meal blood glucose response, you should know which foods contain carbohydrate. Check out Table 2.1 on page 33 for a *general* idea of how much carbohydrate is in each of the different food groups. (More specific examples follow later in the chapter.)

As you see, foods in the Protein group—such as meat, fish, poultry, shellfish (without breading, sauce, or gravy)—are carbohydrate free, as are many fats, including oils, butter, margarine.

When Choosing Carbohydrate-Containing Foods, Stick Close To Nature

It turns out Mother was indeed right when she said "Eat your fruits and vegetables!" But we can expand that to include whole grains, beans, and dairy products too! Choosing nutrient-dense, high-fiber foods whenever possible (See Chapter 8 for more information on fiber)—instead of processed foods with added sodium, fat, and sugars—provides vitamins, minerals, and other healthful substances for relatively few calories.

In general, the more natural a food is, the better it is for you. Consider, for example,

Are Sweet Treats Off Limits?

No, sugary sweet treats are not forbidden, but they do carry a high carbohydrate and calorie content. Sweets should be eaten in moderation, and should be accounted for in your meal plan.

Consider as well that many foods marketed to people with diabetes as "diabetic" foods may contain significant amounts of the sugar fructose (often in the form of agave nectar). Fructose *does* still contribute carbohydrate and calories to those food items, so if you choose to use fructose-sweetened items, incorporate accordingly and in moderation.

The same is true for people with diabetes as for the general public—less sugar is better and it's particularly important to avoid displacing nutrient-dense foods with empty calories from sweets. If you do choose to eat sugar-containing foods, include them in your carbohydrate count (if you're counting carbohydrates) and practice moderation by substituting sweet treats for equal calorie amounts of other carbohydrates; the blood glucose effects should be similar. Do consider that foods high in sugar are generally high in calories. If you choose to work an occasional sweet treat into an overall healthy eating pattern, use caution not to take in too many extra calories.

Are Sugary Beverages Off Limits?

Yes. As for sugary beverages (such as regular soda, lemonade, and fruit drinks), it is best to avoid those. It's widely recommended that people with or at risk for diabetes avoid the use of sugar-sweetened beverages in order to reduce the risk of weight gain and heart disease.

the difference in nutrition between a sweet potato and sweet potato chips. Sticking close to nature, a baked sweet potato is lower in fat, lower in calories, higher in fiber, richer in vitamins and minerals, and more filling than a serving of highly processed potato chips. (And cheaper too!)

It's More Than Just Sugar: Sizing Up Serving Sizes and Total Carbohydrate

If you've already been looking at the nutrition information label on the foods you eat, good for you! (Chapter 4 will give you a full

Table 2.1	Carbohydrate in Foods
Food group (or choice)	**Carbohydrate per serving (grams)**
Starch	15
Fruits	15
Milk and milk substitutes	12
Sweets, desserts, and other carbohydrates	15
Nonstarchy vegetables	5
Proteins	0
Plant-based proteins	Varies
Fats	0
Alcohol	Varies

Academy of Nutrition and Dietetics, American Diabetes Association. *Choose Your Foods: Food Lists for Diabetes.* Chicago, IL, Academy of Nutrition and Dietetics, American Diabetes Association, 2014.

rundown on how to use the information on the nutrition information label.) If not, then it's time to start familiarizing yourself with the serving sizes listed on the labels of your favorite foods and beverages. Compare those serving sizes to the amount of these foods and beverages you normally consume. (Chapter 3 provides tips on portion control and estimated portion sizes.)

Also, when reading nutrition information labels, take a look at the amount of total carbohydrate for the serving size. Many people with diabetes focus just on the sugar content of foods, but sugar is only one type of carbohydrate. Looking only at the grams of sugar does not factor in all of the carbohydrate in the food that will affect your blood glucose. Today, begin refocusing your attention on "Total Carbohydrate" on the nutrition information label, which accounts for all of the carbohydrate in the food. That's the number to use when tallying your carbohydrate count. Many people prefer to track exact grams of carbohydrate. Others prefer to track carbohydrate in terms of carbohydrate choices (servings). Every 15 grams of carbohydrate equals one carbohydrate choice, as noted earlier in this chapter (see "Carbohydrate Counting" on page 29).

Is It True You Need To Subtract Fiber from the Carbohydrate Count?

For most people who are carb counting, it's not necessary to routinely subtract the grams of fiber from the amount of total carbohydrate to lower the total carbohydrate count. See Chapter 8 and Chapter 9 for more information on fiber.

Test Your Carbohydrate Knowledge

Which foods contain carbohydrate?	
Diet soda	
Brown rice	
Orange juice	
Oatmeal	
Watermelon	
Grilled salmon	
Sugar-free ice cream	
Broccoli	
Skim milk	
Olive oil	
Breaded chicken tenders	
Yogurt	

Answer: All contain carbohydrate, except diet soda, grilled salmon, and olive oil.

Step 2: Build Awareness of How Much Carbohydrate You're Eating and Drinking

Admittedly, familiarizing yourself with portion sizes and the associated carbohydrate content of foods and beverages takes some thought and effort, especially in the first few weeks. Chapter 3 provides a multitude of tips to size up your portions both by actually measuring them and by estimation.

To assist in building your carbohydrate awareness, you can keep a carbohydrate count list (whether written, on your computer, or on your smartphone), with the carbohydrate count of portions of your favorite foods for quick reference. Based on our years in practice, we find that most people have around 100 foods and beverages that they routinely consume. Since many people eat the same foods from week to week, our patients often share that they quickly become familiar with the carbohydrate amounts in their favorite foods and beverages. Carbohydrate counting and control become much easier—almost second nature—the more you practice.

There are several resources available to help you quantify the amount of carbohydrate in foods you eat:

- **Nutrition information labels on food and beverage packaging:** This is the most direct source for carbohydrate information. (You'll learn lots about how to understand nutrition information labels in Chapter 4.) Of course, fresh foods, such as apples and broccoli, don't often come with labels. But you can become familiar with the carbohydrate content of these foods through the variety of other resources available.
- **Reliable websites:**
  - *Calorie King* (www.calorieking. com) is a popular website that offers a free, huge, online database that you can search by food or even by specific brands.
  - *USDA National Nutrient Database for Standard Reference* (http://ndb. nal.usda.gov)
  - *SuperTracker* (www.supertracker. usda.gov)
- **Internet search by restaurant for food/beverage names:** Chains and larger establishments often have the nutrition information for their menu items posted online. Many food and beverage manufacturers also post nutrition information of their products on their website.

- **Mobile apps:** MyFitnessPal, for example, is a favorite among our patients.
- **Carbohydrate-counting guidebooks:** Books such as *The Diabetes Carbohydrate & Fat Gram Guide, 4th Edition* and *The Complete Guide to Carb Counting, 3rd Edition* are available from the American Diabetes Association (http://store.diabetes.org).
- *Choose Your Foods: Food Lists for Diabetes* **booklet:** This resource is available from the American Diabetes Association and the Academy of Nutrition and Dietetics (http://store. diabetes.org).

Ask your diabetes educator or registered dietitian/registered dietitian nutritionist for other reputable resources.

Step 3: Know How Much Carbohydrate You Need

Determining the right amount of carbohydrate for you (both per meal/snack and per day) depends on several things, including your:

- Weight
- Height
- Age
- Physical activity
- Food preferences
- Eating patterns
- Diabetes medications (if any)
- Health goals (such as managing blood lipids or weight)

Basic Carbohydrate Goals for Meals and Snacks for Women

As a general starting point, most women need about 45–60 grams of carbohydrate (3–4 carbohydrate choices) at each of their 3 meals and 15 grams for a snack (1 carbohydrate choice). A carbohydrate reduction to 30–45 grams of carbohydrate per meal (2–3 carbohydrate choices) may assist even more with weight loss.

Basic Carbohydrate Goals for Meals and Snacks for Men

As a general starting point, most men need about 60–75 grams of carbohydrate at each meal (4–5 carbohydrate choices) and 15–30 grams for a snack (1–2 carbohydrate choices). To lose weight, a reduction to 45–60 grams of carbohydrate (3–4 carbohydrate choices) per meal can help.

Carbohydrate Control Is Like Using a Checking Account

Think about carbohydrate control like this— your meal and snack carbohydrate goals are like a checking account. At each meal, you have roughly 45–60 grams of carbohydrate (or 60–75 grams of carbohydrate) in your account to "spend." You can spend it on whichever carbohydrate-containing foods you wish. There are generally no "forbidden" foods, but you may find that you end up eating smaller portions of certain foods and eating some foods less often. While not the healthiest choice, you can even have an occasional splurge, like a chocolate donut, if you plan ahead and allocate grams of carbohydrate to spend on it. Of course, the goal is to spend the majority of your carbohydrate grams on a variety of healthy foods. If you "overdraw" your carbohydrate account, the "penalty" is that your blood glucose will run higher after the meal. The same rules apply for snacks.

How Much Carbohydrate Do You Need?*

Women	Men
Women should have about **45–60 grams** of carbohydrate at each of three meals and **15 grams** for one snack (if your health-care team advises you to have snacks).	Men should have about **60–75 grams** of carbohydrate at each of three meals and **15–30 grams** for one snack (if your health-care team advises you to have snacks).
That's 150–195 grams of carbohydrate over the whole day.	That's 195–255 grams of carbohydrate over the whole day.

*For growing children/teens, carbohydrate needs may vary significantly to support growth and activity. These general guidelines are intended to apply to adults. Discuss your individual carbohydrate needs with your health-care team.

Keep in mind that this approach does not allow you to reserve or save carbohydrate from one meal or snack to "spend" on a later meal or snack (unless you are instructed by your health-care team to follow advanced insulin matching rules). There is no savings account. Use it or lose it. So, spend your carbohydrate wisely to work in those foods that you enjoy!

Once you meet with a registered dietitian nutritionist and/or your health-care team, they can refine your carbohydrate goals for meals and snacks if necessary.

Rate Your Plate

After you create your plate (a 9-inch plate is the perfect size to use), whether you're at the work potluck, church social, restaurant buffet, or in your own kitchen, take a close look at the foods and portions you've put on your plate. Then answer the following questions:

- **Is about 1/4 of your plate filled with a starchy vegetable, grain, or beans?**
  That's about 30–45 grams of carbohydrate or 2–3 carbohydrate choices.
- **Is about 1/4 of your plate filled with a protein food, such as lean meat, poultry, or fish?**
  That's carbohydrate free—unless it's breaded or has a carbohydrate-containing sauce/accompaniment.
- **Is at least 1/2 of your plate filled with nonstarchy vegetables?**
  That's about 10–15 grams of carbohydrate or about 1 carbohydrate choice.
- **Do you have a serving of fruit and/or a cup of milk or milk substitute on the side to balance your plate (as your meal plan allows)?**
  The fruit adds 15 grams of carbohydrate or 1 carbohydrate choice. The milk/milk substitute adds another 12 grams of carbohydrate or 1 carbohydrate choice.
- **Is your plate colorful?**

See "Create Your Plate" in Chapter 1 for additional guidelines. **The goal is to be able to answer "Yes" to all of the questions above. How did your plate stack up?** Fill your plate in this manner to help control your carbohydrate intake and ensure that you're getting variety, a good balance of nutrients, and controlled portions.

Mexican Meal Carbohydrate Conundrum

Suppose you are eating at a Mexican restaurant and find yourself in this scenario:

You order two beef-and-cheese tacos with a side of refried beans and rice. As you wait for the food, you munch your way through half a basket of tortilla chips and salsa while sipping on a margarita. After all, it is happy hour! How does the carbohydrate in this meal stack up? Put your carbohydrate-counting skills to work, and decide what to do.

Carbohydrate goal: 60–75 grams for the meal

Food	Portion	Carbohydrate (grams)
ALREADY EATEN		
Chips & salsa	12 chips + 1/4 cup salsa	20
Margarita	6 ounces	25
TOTAL SO FAR: 45		
STILL TO COME		
Beef and cheese tacos	2	26
Refried beans	1/2 cup	15
Mexican rice	1/2 cup	25
TOTAL TO COME: 66		
GRAND TOTAL: 111		

What Should You Do?

If you eat all of this meal, in addition to the chips and margarita, your carbohydrate intake will total 111 grams—or nearly double your mealtime goal. Oops! Because you've already eaten 45 grams of carbohydrate, you could eat just half of the meal (for 33 grams of carbohydrate) to get a grand total of 78 grams of carbohydrate. Box up the rest of the meal, and take it home for lunch tomorrow. Although 78 grams of carbohydrate is slightly above your target of 60–75 grams, it's still very close.

A Few Other Carbohydrate Considerations

"Free" Doesn't Always Mean Free

Although some sugar-free foods, such as diet soda, are truly sugar free, carbohydrate free, and calorie free, most sugar-free foods still have calories, fat, and carbohydrate. "Sugar free" means simply that no sugar or sugar-based sweetener has been added to the food or beverage. "Sugar free" does not necessarily mean that the food is carbohydrate free or calorie free.

Often, "sugar-free" foods, such as sugar-free chocolates, contain a special type of sweetener called "sugar alcohols." You may find the amount of sugar alcohols listed on the nutrition information label. You can check the ingredient list for sugar alcohols as well (see "Common Sugar Alcohols"). Be aware that these sweeteners *do* contain carbohydrate and *will* affect your blood glucose, although to a lesser extent than sugar. They may have a laxative effect, too, causing intestinal bloating, gas, and diarrhea.

Remember to check out the grams of total carbohydrate on the nutrition information label to see just how much carbohydrate is in a food or beverage. You might be surprised by what you find.

Common Sugar Alcohols

- Erythritol
- Glycerol
- Hydrogenated starch hydrolysates
- Isomalt
- Lactitol
- Maltitol
- Mannitol
- Sorbitol
- Xylitol

Remember, sugar alcohols can raise your blood glucose! Check your blood glucose 1 1/2–2 hours after eating sugar alcohol–containing food to note the effect it has on you.

Is It True You Need to Subtract Sugar Alcohols from the Carbohydrate Count?

If you've heard about subtracting sugar alcohols from carbohydrate count, you may be wondering, "What's the story?" If a food contains >5 grams of sugar alcohols per serving, you *can* subtract half of the grams of sugar alcohol from the total carbohydrate grams to reduce the total carbohydrate grams (since sugar alcohols affect blood glucose less than sugar). For most people, though, it's not necessary to do that extra math.

See Chapter 9 for more information on sugar alcohols.

The Scoop on Chocolate Ice Cream

A 1/2-cup serving of regular chocolate ice cream contains 18 grams of total carbohydrate, whereas the same size serving of fat-free, no-sugar-added chocolate ice cream has *even more* grams of total carbohydrate—26 grams! You might have thought that the no-sugar-added ice cream would be a low-carbohydrate choice. Not so. The unexpected carbohydrate comes from sugar alcohols.

As this example illustrates, "sugar free" definitely does not mean "carbohydrate free." Sugar-free foods can be part of a diabetes meal plan as long as you count the carbohydrate accordingly. Talk further with your registered dietitian nutritionist or certified diabetes educator about how sugar alcohols can fit into your meal plan.

Low-Calorie Sweeteners: A Personal Choice

Blue, pink, yellow, green, orange—such is the rainbow of packaging colors for the variety of low-calorie sweeteners available today. These sweeteners are also called "high-intensity sweeteners," "non-nutritive sweeteners," "sugar substitutes," or "artificial sweeteners" (although the stevia and monk fruit sweeteners you'll see in "Low-Calorie Sweeteners Available in the U.S." are not artificial; they come from plant extracts). See Chapter 9 for more information on low-calorie (non-nutritive) sweeteners. Only a relatively small amount of a low-calorie sweetener is needed because they are several hundred to several thousand times sweeter than sugar. These sweeteners are different from sugar alcohols.

Use of low-calorie sweeteners is a personal choice for people with diabetes. Low-calorie sweeteners provide sweetness with nearly no carbohydrate or calories, meaning they don't impact blood glucose; however, other ingredients in a food or beverage containing low-calorie sweeteners may in fact affect blood glucose. For instance, sugar-free, fruit-flavored yogurt contains a low-calorie sweetener but still has 12 grams of carbohydrate per 6-ounce cup, on average. An additional consideration is that while low-calorie sweetener use has the potential to reduce overall calorie and carbohydrate intake, that's true only if they're *substituted* for caloric sweetener without compensating by eating additional calories elsewhere.

There are currently eight low-calorie sweeteners available in the U.S. The U.S. Food and Drug Administration (FDA) has approved six low-calorie sweeteners for use in the U.S. The monk fruit and stevia low-calorie sweeteners have Generally Recognized as Safe (GRAS) status.

If you choose to use a low-calorie sweetener and don't like the taste of the first one you try, switch to another. You may prefer the taste of one over another. Or, if you choose to refrain from using low-calorie sweeteners altogether and stick with a sugar-sweetened versions of your favorite foods/beverages, just know that the carbohydrate content of the

Low-Calorie Sweeteners Available in the U.S.*

- Acesulfame potassium or Ace-K for short (Sweet One)
- Advantame
- Aspartame (Equal, Nutrasweet)
- Monk fruit extract or Luo Han Guo (Purefruit)
- Neotame (Newtame)
- Saccharin (Sweet'N Low, Sugar Twin)
- Stevia (PureVia, Truvia)
- Sucralose (Splenda)

Store-brand versions of these sweeteners may be available in your local store.

"regular" versions will be higher. You'll have to "spend" more carbohydrate to fit it in.

As for safety, low-calorie sweeteners and sugar alcohols are considered safe when consumed within the daily intake levels established by the FDA. If you're concerned about sugar alcohols and low-calorie sweeteners, talk with your registered dietitian nutritionist or diabetes educator.

What about Glycemic Index and Glycemic Load?

Glycemic Index

You may have read about glycemic index (GI) and glycemic load (GL), or seen an advertisement touting the benefits of low GI/GL foods. While some organizations may suggest the use of a low-GI diet, research shows that GI and GL in relation to diabetes are complex because

blood glucose response to a particular food varies among individuals and can be impacted by a number of factors.

The GI is a method that ranks carbohydrates on a scale from 0–100 according to how they raise blood glucose after eating. (See "Glycemic Index Rankings.")

- **Low-GI foods** produce gradual rises in blood glucose levels because they are slowly digested and absorbed.
- **High-GI foods** are rapidly digested and absorbed and lead to marked elevations in blood glucose.

Two foods having the same carbohydrate content in grams, may have differing glycemic index rankings or glycemic loads.

Jelly Beans vs. Kidney Beans

For example, if you have one serving of jelly beans and one of kidney beans, and both portions have the same carbohydrate content, the jelly beans will be digested more rapidly and raise your blood glucose more than kidney beans. In other words, jelly beans have a higher GI than kidney beans. Of course, to deliver the same carbohydrate amount, the portion sizes of these two foods would be different.

To complicate matters further, the GI of a specific food can change based on a number of factors including what else is eaten during the meal or with the food, how the food is processed and prepared, the acidity, fat content, and fiber content of the food, and many other factors. Even factors unrelated to the food can affect the GI, such as time of day, mealtime blood glucose level, stress, and the physical fitness of the individual.

Glycemic Load

"But what about portion size?" you may ask. "What if I'm eating a bite of cheesecake, not a whole slice? Does that matter?" The GI of a food does not change whether you eat a bite of cheesecake or an entire slice. Eating a larger amount of a carbohydrate-containing food

---

Glycemic Index Rankings

Understanding glycemic index rankings can be difficult. Here is a breakdown to help you understand what GI numbers indicate.

- Low GI: 55 or less
- Moderate GI: 56–69
- High GI: 70 or higher

Do you want to know the glycemic index of a favorite food?

Check out the online database at www.glycemicindex.com.

If some of your favorite foods are high GI, you may be able to trade them for lower-GI versions. See the examples below.

High–glycemic index favorites	Lower–glycemic index trade-off
French bread: 81	Stoneground whole-wheat bread: 59
Baked white potato, no skin: 98	Boiled yam, no skin: 35
Pretzels: 83	Popcorn: 55

Here is a breakdown to help you understand what GL numbers mean:

Glycemic Load Rankings
- Low GL: 10 or less
- Moderate GL: 11–19
- High GL: 20 or higher

(such as a *slice* of cheesecake) will certainly raise your blood glucose more than eating a smaller amount (a *bite* of cheesecake, for example). That's where glycemic load (GL) comes into the picture. GL takes into account the portion size and potential impact on blood glucose. Substituting low-GL foods for higher-GL foods may modestly improve blood glucose control. A searchable GL database is available at www.glycemicindex.com.

The Bottom Line on GI and GL

The GI and GL are tools that may help you fine-tune your blood glucose levels. The simplest approach to incorporating GI and GL is to choose foods with a lower GI and substitute low-GL foods for high-GL foods, when possible, while still being mindful of the portions you eat. It's up to you whether you'd like to use these tools. Just keep in mind that a food's effect on blood glucose may vary from person to person.

Meeting Your Registered Dietitian/Registered Dietitian Nutritionist and/or Certified Diabetes Educator

For more assistance and guidance on incorporating the carbohydrate foods you enjoy into your eating pattern in amounts that fit your personal health needs, consult with a registered dietitian/registered dietitian nutritionist (RD/RDN) who specializes in diabetes nutrition.

An RD/RDN may provide additional counsel on how to incorporate physical activity into your life as well. For a referral to an RD/RDN, ask your physician or locate one near you through the Academy of Nutrition and Dietetics website (www.eatright.org). Many RD/RDNs are also certified diabetes educators (CDE), and they can help you understand how any diabetes medicines you're taking affect you, teach you how to monitor your blood glucose, and teach you how to solve problems and adjust emotionally to diabetes. For a referral to a certified diabetes educator, ask your physician or locate one through the American Association of Diabetes Educators website (www.diabeteseducator.org) or the National Certification Board for Diabetes Educators website (www.ncbde.org). To make the most of your time and the visit, review the checklist that follows in "Preparing for Your Visit" and take this information to your appointment.

Preparing for Your Visit

If you are newly diagnosed with diabetes, three or four visits to a registered dietitian/registered dietitian nutritionist or certified diabetes educator can help get your diabetes meal plan on track. After that, you should at least have an annual follow-up to help you stay on track.

Here's what to take with you on your visit:

	Consult/referral form from your doctor's office
	Copy of the results from your most recent checkup
	Recent medical and lab tests
	Blood glucose meter, if you have one
	Your blood glucose logbook, if you have been checking your blood glucose at home
	List of all medicines and supplements you take, including the dosages
	Any diet information you have received in the past or are currently following
	Any diabetes/nutrition information that you have been reading or researching
	A food journal (written or electronic) that lists everything you eat and drink in the 3–7 days before the appointment. Remember to include serving sizes and how the food was prepared. Record carbohydrate content, if possible.
	Nutrition information labels on products you have questions about
	A list of questions you want answered
	A report on your progress (if it's a return visit)
	A list of goals you hope to accomplish
	A friend or family member to help provide information and absorb the new information
	Your insurance card and photo identification

Next Steps

- Contact a registered dietitian/registered dietitian nutritionist and/or diabetes educator to schedule an appointment.
- Review the "Preparing for Your Visit" checklist, and gather the information before your appointment.
- Begin compiling a list of favorite foods and carbohydrate counts of portions you frequently eat.

What Do I Eat for Breakfast?

FOR 45–60 GRAMS OF CARBOHYDRATE*

Recipe: Quick Cranberry-Cherry Walnut Oatmeal (1 serving)

1 (1-ounce) link turkey sausage

1 slice whole-wheat toast

1 teaspoon trans fat–free margarine

Coffee or hot tea (with low-calorie sweetener if desired)

1 cup low-fat milk

FOR 60–75 GRAMS OF CARBOHYDRATE*

Recipe: Quick Cranberry-Cherry Walnut Oatmeal (1 serving)

1 (1-ounce) link turkey sausage

2 slices whole-wheat toast

2 teaspoons trans fat–free margarine

Coffee or hot tea (with low-calorie sweetener if desired)

1 cup low-fat milk

For most women, 45–60 grams of carbohydrate at a meal is a good starting point; for most men, 60–75 grams of carbohydrate per meal is appropriate. Check with your diabetes health-care team to find the amount of carbohydrate that's right for you.

Swift, Simple Tip

- Buy ready-to-serve, precooked turkey sausage to heat in the microwave.

QUICK CRANBERRY-CHERRY WALNUT OATMEAL

SERVES: 1

SERVING SIZE: About 1 cup

PREPARATION TIME: 3 minutes

COOKING TIME: 1 1/2–2 minutes

INGREDIENTS

1 (1-ounce) packet plain instant oatmeal

2/3 cup diet cranberry-cherry juice

2 dashes cinnamon

2 teaspoons ground flax seed

1 tablespoon chopped walnuts

1. Empty oatmeal into a microwave-safe bowl. Stir in juice and cinnamon. Microwave uncovered on high power for 1 1/2–2 minutes, or until oatmeal starts to thicken (water or additional juice can be used to thin oatmeal if desired).

2. Stir and sprinkle with flax seed then walnuts. Serve right away.

Recipe Tips

- Buy ground (milled) flax seed. It's often located in the baking ingredients aisle at regular grocery stores. Flax seed boosts the fiber and adds heart-healthy omega-3 fats.
- Buy chopped walnuts.

CHOICES/EXCHANGES

1 1/2 Starch, 1 1/2 Fat

BASIC NUTRITIONAL VALUES

Calories	190	**Potassium**	185 mg
Calories from Fat	80	**Total Carbohydrate**	23 g
Total Fat	9.0 g	Dietary Fiber	5 g
Saturated Fat	1.0 g	Sugars	3 g
Trans Fat	0.0 g	**Protein**	6 g
Cholesterol	0 mg	**Phosphorus**	185 mg
Sodium	130 mg		

Food for Thought

- **Carbohydrate counts most.** Carbohydrate in foods and beverages impacts your blood glucose levels, so familiarize yourself with the total carbohydrate content of your favorite foods and beverages.
- **Keep carbohydrate consistent.** Try to eat and drink about the same amount of carbohydrate at meals and snacks each day to stabilize your blood glucose.
- **Most foods can fit.** You can work in and enjoy nearly any food if you count the carbohydrate and fit it into your meal or snack carbohydrate goals.
- **Balance your plate.** When serving your plate, try to keep it colorful and fill half of the plate with nonstarchy vegetables, one-fourth with lean meat/poultry/fish, and one-fourth with starchy vegetables, grains, or starchy beans. Round it out with a piece of fruit and a cup of milk/milk substitute if your plan allows it.
- **Enjoy your food.** Choose carbohydrate foods you enjoy in amounts that fit your carbohydrate goals, so you can feel satisfied.

Portion Distortion: Have You Encountered It?

Have you ever found yourself thinking, "I can't believe I ate the whole thing!"? It's no secret that portion sizes in the U.S. have inflated over the years. Consider twenty years ago . . .

1. A bagel was 3 inches in diameter and 140 calories; now the average bagel is 6 inches in diameter and 350 calories.
    An average man of 5′ 10″ weighing about 155 pounds would have to play basketball for 30 minutes to burn off the extra 210 calories!
2. A standard serving of french fries was 2.4 ounces and 210 calories; now it's nearly double that, at about 5 ounces and 410 calories.
    That same average man of 5′ 10″ weighing about 155 pounds would have to do 75 minutes of light yard work to burn off those 410 calories!

Consumers' perception of appropriate portion sizes has become distorted over time, with larger portions now viewed as the normal appropriate amount to eat on a single occasion. Food portions are larger than they were 20 years ago at almost every food venue, from markets to vending machines to restaurants.

Super-sizing your order or going to an "all you can eat" buffet may seem like a bargain for your wallet, but is it really a bargain if your blood glucose is too high 2 hours later? Diving into a bowl of macaroni and cheese or pasta may bring you comfort in the moment, but are tight clothes or high blood glucose comfortable later on? Slicing off a large piece of cake or pie may seem sweet at the time, but is the high blood glucose and sluggishness that hits a few hours later so sweet?

Why the Concern about Portion Size?

Portion sizes are a big concern because larger portions mean more calories, more carbohydrate, and thus a greater impact on blood glucose levels and weight. Weight management is a concern for many people with type 2 diabetes. According to the American Diabetes Association's "Nutrition Therapy Recommendations for the Management of Adults with Diabetes," more than 3 out of 4 adults with diabetes are at least "overweight" (BMI 25–29.9) In fact, nearly half of all those with diabetes actually fall into the obese category (BMI ≥30). Because extra body fat is linked to insulin resistance, and thus blood glucose control challenges, weight loss has long been a recommended strategy for overweight or obese adults with diabetes. Prevention of weight gain is equally important.

Build Awareness of Portion Sizes

Nutrition Information

A growing positive trend is the increasing availability of nutrition information—from the label on food packages to calorie content and other nutrition information at the point of purchase—with the intent to raise consumer awareness and allow you make to informed decisions. Do compare the portion you actually eat to the serving size associated with the nutrition information. If you eat double the serving size noted, then double the calorie, carbohydrate, and other nutrient counts too.

Has seeing the calorie count posted on menus and food packages changed your food and beverage decisions?

Dish and Glass Size

Just as portion sizes have increased, so have the sizes of dishes and glasses. People used to drink juice from 4-ounce juice glasses. Now 10- to 16-ounce glasses and 25-ounce tumblers are typical. No longer is eating on 9-inch plates the norm. Now plates are 11–12 inches or larger. Because a "normal"-size portion looks small in a large glass or on a large plate, people tend to over-serve when using larger glasses and plates. Research confirms that people eat and drink more when they're served larger portions.

Package Size

"Individual serving" packages may not always be healthy single-serving portions. In some

Using Larger Dishes = Larger Portions = More Calories = Weight Gain

Did You Know . . .

Reducing your plate size from 12 inches to 10 inches results in 22% fewer calories being served on average? Based on this percentage, if a typical dinner has 800 calories, using a smaller plate would lead to a weight loss of around 18 pounds per year for an average-size adult.[1]

instances the serving in those packages may be much more than you actually need. **Studies show that the bigger the package you pour from, the more you will eat—20 to 30% more for most foods.**

Are a Few Extra Pounds a Concern for You?

Whether you desire to drop a few pounds or proactively prevent weight gain, **reducing calories while maintaining a healthful eating pattern is the bottom line**. And as reviewed in Chapter 1, you're not locked into any one "ideal diet" to accomplish that goal; a variety of eating patterns can achieve calorie and glucose control. Many studies have shown the Mediterranean style of eating leads to the greatest weight loss; however, you may also achieve weight-management success via a low-fat or low-carbohydrate eating pattern,

through a vegetarian or vegan eating pattern, or through the DASH (Dietary Approaches to Stop Hypertension) eating style. Total calorie intake, and thus portion sizes, are an important consideration no matter which eating pattern you go with.

Size Up Your Portions— Do You Eat More Than You Think?

As famous actor, director, writer, and producer Orson Welles once quipped: "My doctor told me to stop having intimate dinners for four. Unless there are three other people." The key message here is to take a look at your portions and size them up. What you may currently think of as a "regular" portion size may not, in fact, be the "best for you" portion size. Are your portions too large, too small, or just right?

---

[1] Wansink B, Roizen M. *Mindless Dieting: Newsletter #1 of a Series* [Internet]. Available from http://mindlesseating.org/pdf/Mindless_Dieting_01.pdf

> **Think 20% Less**
>
> Most often, people can eat 20% less without noticing it. Serve up 20% less than you think you might want before you start to eat.

Practical Methods and Tools to Size Up Portions

Many people think they eat less than they actually do. In fact, studies show that people tend to underestimate the calories in large meals—the larger the meal, the more the calorie estimation is off. As for carbohydrate control, becoming familiar with serving sizes can help you pinpoint how much you actually eat and whether you are meeting or exceeding your meal and snack carbohydrate goals.

How much does your cereal bowl hold? Is it 1 cup? Or is it actually closer to 2 or 3 cups?

Going one step further, keep track of the actual portion sizes of what you eat (see the following three approaches to determining portion sizes). You may choose to track your food, beverages, and portions through a written log, a mobile app, online, or on the computer—whatever method works for you. And even if you can't track it every day, any information is better than none. We bet you'll make some enlightening discoveries.

There are three approaches that you can use to determine portion sizes.

Approach #1: Measuring Tools

The most accurate way to monitor portion sizes is to measure your food or beverage with measuring cups, measuring spoons, or a food scale. Be sure to use liquid measuring cups for liquids

---

3 Approaches to Determine Portion Sizes

#1 Measuring tools (measuring cups, spoons, scales)
- *Example:* Weigh a chicken breast on a food scale to identify a 3-ounce portion.

#2 Hand estimations (using your hand as a guide to estimate portion sizes)
- *Example:* Compare a chicken breast to the palm of your hand. Three ounces is about the size of a woman's palm, and five ounces is the size of a man's palm.

#3 Comparison of food portions to common household items
- *Example:* Three ounces of chicken breast is about the size of a deck of cards.

You may choose to utilize all 3 of these approaches at one time or another to help you estimate and stay in touch with portion sizes.

Top Tips for Measuring Portions

- **Measure your drinking cups.** Fill your drinking cups with water, and then pour it into a liquid measuring cup to determine how many ounces your cups hold. You'll then know how much you drink when you fill the cup all the way or just part of the way.
- **Measure your bowls.** Fill your bowls with dry cereal and then measure the cereal with a dry measuring cup to identify how much the bowls hold and how much you eat when you fill them up.
- **Measure your plate.** Is it a 9-inch plate? Or more like 11–12 inches?
- **Use a measuring cup to serve foods (such as soup, vegetables, casserole, or cereal) rather than using a spoon or ladle.** You can then easily quantify the amount you eat, and thus determine the carbohydrate count. We gleaned this tip from a patient years ago, and it is now a favorite practice among many of our patients.
- **When possible, measure out appropriate individual portions of foods.** For instance, use a measuring cup to put leftover casserole or chili into small plastic containers for reheating. Or measure appropriate portions of cereal or snacks and store them in zip-top plastic bags. That way, no thinking is required when you go to grab the leftovers for lunch or a snack.

and dry measuring cups for non-liquids—there is a difference. Most people are surprised to see how their actual portion sizes measure up against what they "thought" they were eating.

Try this at home . . .

- Over the next couple of weeks, try to measure your food portions as often as possible. The more you actually weigh and measure food, the better you will get at eyeballing portion sizes. You'll soon become familiar with what 1/2 cup of beans looks like on your plate, what 8 ounces of milk looks like in

a glass, and what 1 cup of high-fiber breakfast cereal looks like in a bowl.

- Once a month, do a spot check to make sure you're still visualizing your portion sizes correctly.

Approach #2: Hand Estimations

Although measuring cups and spoons certainly have their place, they aren't always convenient or even realistic to use on many eating occasions. (Who wants to take measuring cups to a friend's house for dinner? Or to the deli at lunch?) In those scenarios, rely on your own hand to estimate portion sizes and carbohydrate counts using the "Handy Guidelines for Portion Estimation" below.

If you use the handy guidelines when you visit a steakhouse, you may find that the steak you ordered is about 10 ounces (two man-sized palms) and that the side of potatoes is about 1 cup (a small adult fist).

Should you order spaghetti in a restaurant, you can quickly determine the portion size on the plate. Typically the plate arrives with at least 2 cups of cooked spaghetti (that's 2 small adult fists' worth). Knowing that 1/3 cup cooked spaghetti has 15 grams of carbohydrate (or 1 carbohydrate choice), you'll realize that a 2-cup plate of spaghetti contains a whopping 90 grams of carbohydrate (or 6 carbohydrate choices)! No wonder many people notice

their blood glucose is above target after eating spaghetti—the portion size is just too large.

When you go to a dinner party, using your hand as a guide, you can select a 3-ounce piece of grilled chicken breast (size of the a woman's palm), a teaspoon of margarine (1 thumb tip) for your roll, and 2 tablespoons (2 thumbs) of dressing for your salad.

Approach #3: Visualize the Right Portion Size

Another method to help you become familiar with portion sizes is to compare them with everyday household items. Some of our favorite comparisons are on the next page; you may come up with others that work for you.

Once you gain familiarity with standard portion sizes, you can easily compare them to

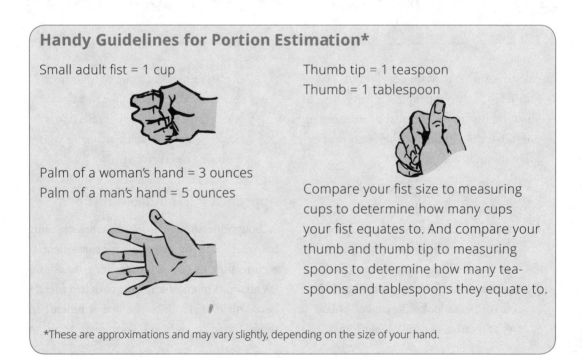

Handy Guidelines for Portion Estimation*

Small adult fist = 1 cup

Palm of a woman's hand = 3 ounces
Palm of a man's hand = 5 ounces

Thumb tip = 1 teaspoon
Thumb = 1 tablespoon

Compare your fist size to measuring cups to determine how many cups your fist equates to. And compare your thumb and thumb tip to measuring spoons to determine how many teaspoons and tablespoons they equate to.

*These are approximations and may vary slightly, depending on the size of your hand.

Household Item Estimations

Portion size	Common item
3 ounces meat	Deck of cards
2 tablespoons peanut butter	Ping pong ball
1 ounce cheese	Domino, lipstick, or 4 dice
1/2 medium bagel	Hockey puck
Small potato	Computer mouse
1/2 cup vegetables	Light bulb
Medium-size piece of fruit	Tennis ball

the amount you eat and then calculate how many grams of carbohydrate are in your portions. You will quickly become confident and competent at experience-based estimation of portions and their associated carbohydrate content.

Become an Illusionist: Smaller Dishes Equal "Larger" Portions

Make visual tricks work for you by using smaller dishes to make portions appear larger, and thus trick your mind into believing you're getting larger portions than you are. Here are some examples of how to trick your mind using plate and glass sizes:

- Plate size: 1 cup of black beans and rice on an 8-inch plate appears to be a nice size serving. However, 1 cup on a 12-inch plate looks like a little appetizer. The illusion of the "larger"

portion on the 8-inch plate will likely leave you feeling more satisfied.

- Glass size: With glasses, think slender. A tall, slender 8-ounce glass makes your beverage portion appear larger than it would in a short, wide 8-ounce glass. If you don't fill your glass all the way, studies show you'll tend to pour 30% more into a wide glass than you would into a slender one.

Preportion to Head Off Portion Distortion

Another strategy to manage portion sizes, and control the temptation to overeat, is to incorporate preportioned foods whenever possible. Whether you choose to purchase items preportioned, or portion them out yourself into zip-top bags or individual containers at home is up to you. Have a favorite combination of

More Tips to Manage Portion Size

Eating out	Split an entrée or meal with your dining companion.
	Ask for a to-go box with your meal and pack up half the entrée (or meal) before you begin eating.
	Request a "lunch size" or "half" portion.
	Order a kid's meal.
	Try a small appetizer or soup plus a side salad in place of a larger meal.
Eating in	Use smaller dishes and more slender glasses, so that you eat less but your portions appear larger.
	Serve from the stove, so you're not tempted to eat more than your portion; if the food is out of reach, then you won't be as tempted to get "just a little bit more."
Eating between meals	Keep preportioned snacks available in amounts that fit your carbohydrate goals (whether you buy them preportioned or do the work yourself).
	See what you eat by serving a portion that matches your carbohydrate and calorie needs in a bowl or container. Resist snacking from the bag or package because it's much more difficult to know how much you've eaten.

What about Meal Replacements?

A meal replacement is a drink, bar, or shake intended to be used as a substitute for a meal. They usually have controlled quantities of calories, carbohydrate, and other nutrients. Meal replacements can be valuable if you choose to use them occasionally when you just don't want to think or make a decision about what or how much to eat. They're portion controlled, and it's easy to glance at the label and see exactly what nutrients and how much carbohydrate you're getting. Keep a few meal replacements on hand that fit your calorie, carbohydrate, and health needs.

> **"View It before You Chew It"**
>
> Put everything you eat in a separate dish before you start eating so you can see exactly how much you're eating and make adjustments as needed to achieve your carbohydrate target. Leave the package, bag, or container in the kitchen and you'll be less likely to go back for more.

snack mix ingredients? Portion out "right-for-you," carbohydrate-controlled portions that are ready to grab and go. Preportioned foods means no thinking required when hunger hits.

Here are a few examples of preportioned foods you may enjoy:

- fresh apple, orange, pear, plum
- instant oatmeal packets
- 100-calorie snack packs (such as 100-calorie packs of almonds)
- individual greek yogurt cups
- Laughing Cow or Babybel Light individual light snack cheeses
- individual snack packs of hummus, baby carrots, or apple slices
- healthy, natural frozen meals

Make Swaps to Save Calories Where You Can: Small Calorie Savings Add Up

Granted, trimming portions automatically trims calories. But small switches in the *types* of foods you eat and beverages you drink can save calories yet still satisfy your appetite and taste buds.

If you are trying to cut a few calories in order to trim a few pounds, saving just 300 calories a day means 2100 fewer calories to worry about at the week's end. And saving 500 calories a day means 3500 calories less at week's end. No doubt that's a step in the right direction!

In the end, almost any food can fit in your diabetes meal plan in moderation. Moderation is the mantra—the key is how much of a food you eat and how often you eat it.

Embrace Mindful Eating

Mindful eating means slowing down, being aware and mindful of what and how much you eat, and really tasting and savoring the food. **Most people find that the first two to three bites bring the most pleasure.** After that, what they eat is just "noise" and they don't really enjoy or need any more.

Two- to Three-Bite Taste Test

Try the two- to three-bite taste test yourself! Read on to see how it works ...

A patient we've worked with in the past loved cheesecake. Prior to developing diabetes she'd eat an entire giant slice when she dined at her favorite restaurant. Once diabetes entered her life, she still wanted to try to work in cheesecake on occasion, and realized that portion control was important. We had her try the two- to three-bite taste test. She reported back that she discovered she really savored the first three bites of her cheesecake, but after that the pleasure decreased. Based on her discovery, she decided to eat just three bites of cheesecake at the meal, count and incorporate the carbohydrate accordingly,

---

Calorie Swap Examples

7 Swaps to Save 100 Calories*

- Enjoy a small (4-ounce) orange rather than 12 ounces of natural orange juice.
- Sip on a "tall" (12-ounce) "skinny" mocha coffee drink instead of the regular version.
- Nestle your lunchtime sandwich between 2 slice of light whole-wheat bread instead of regular bread.
- Drizzle 3 tablespoons vinaigrette on your salad rather than creamy dressing.
- Pick a cup of pears canned in juice over those canned in heavy syrup.
- Savor a spring roll over a fried egg roll.
- Steam veggies and top with a light drizzle of olive oil rather than sautéing in oil.

7 Swaps to Save 200 Calories*

- Pack flavor in your omelet with 1/4 cup onions and peppers rather than 1/4 cup shredded cheese.
- Choose a thin bagel in place of a large traditional bagel.
- Go for 4 ounces of grilled fish instead of fried.
- Dunk a cup of cucumber slices in your salsa rather than 18–20 tortilla chips.
- Crush the chocolate craving with a no-sugar-added frozen fudge pop over 1 cup of chocolate ice cream.
- Choose 1 cup mashed cauliflower over buttery mashed potatoes.
- Munch 2 slices of a medium veggie pizza instead of "the meats" pizza.

Use a few of these swaps in one day, and you'll save 300–500 calories!

*Calorie savings are approximate (plus/minus 25 calories).

and take the rest home to spread out the pleasure (and carbohydrate) by enjoying two to three bites at several more meals.

For additional guidance and support when it comes managing your portions, stay in frequent contact with your diabetes health-care team, particularly your registered dietitan/registered dietitian nutritionist. That frequent contact, ongoing education, counseling, and support is important for consistent and sustained weight loss.

Next Steps

Pull out your measuring cups, measuring spoons, and food scale, and let the fun begin!

- Measure 1 cup of cold cereal. Pour it into a bowl and notice how it fills the bowl.
- Weigh a potato that is the size you usually eat.
- Measure 1/3 cup of cooked rice or pasta. Place it on your plate, and compare that with how much pasta or rice you usually eat.
- Measure 8 ounces of milk in a liquid measuring cup. Pour it into a drinking glass, and note how much it fills the glass.
- Measure 4 ounces of juice in a liquid measuring cup. Pour it into a glass, and note how much it fills the glass.
- Weigh an apple, orange, or banana that is the size you usually eat.
- Measure 1/2 cup of green beans or another vegetable. Place them on your plate, and compare that with how much your typical vegetable portion fills the plate.
- Measure 1 tablespoon of salad dressing. Drizzle it over lettuce, and notice how that compares with the amount of dressing you usually put on salads.
- Measure out 2 tablespoons of nuts and then 1/4 cup of nuts. Note how those amounts compare to the portion you usually eat.

What Do I Eat for Dinner?

FOR 45–60 GRAMS OF CARBOHYDRATE*
3 ounces grilled shrimp
Recipe: Mediterranean Quinoa Salad (1 cup)
1 cup steamed asparagus topped with a light
    drizzle of olive oil and a squeeze of fresh
    lemon
1 1/2 cups diced watermelon

FOR 60–75 GRAMS OF CARBOHYDRATE*
3 ounces grilled shrimp
Recipe: Mediterranean Quinoa Salad (1 cup)
1 cup steamed asparagus topped with a light
    drizzle of olive oil and a squeeze of fresh
    lemon
1/2 (6-inch) whole-wheat pita bread
1 1/2 cups diced watermelon

*For most women, 45–60 grams of carbohydrate at a meal is a good starting point; for most men, 60–75 grams of carbohydrate per meal is appropriate. Check with your diabetes health-care team to find the amount of carbohydrate that's right for you.

Swift, Simple Tips

- As an alternative to grilling shrimp, buy fully cooked shrimp and stir into the Mediterranean Quinoa Salad.
- Buy steam-in-the-bag asparagus cuts.

MEDITERRANEAN QUINOA SALAD

SERVES: 5

SERVING SIZE: 1 cup

PREPARATION TIME: 30 minutes

COOKING TIME: 15 minutes

INGREDIENTS FOR SALAD

1 cup uncooked quinoa

2 cups low-sodium chicken broth

1 cup cherry tomatoes, halved

1 cup diced cucumber

1/2 cup canned chickpeas, drained and rinsed

1/2 cup kalamata olives, chopped

1/2 cup reduced-fat feta cheese

1 tablespoon chopped fresh mint

2 tablespoons chopped fresh parsley

INGREDIENTS FOR DRESSING

1 tablespoon olive oil

Juice of 1 lemon

1 clove garlic, minced or grated

1. Rinse uncooked quinoa thoroughly in a fine strainer under cold running water until water runs clear. Combine quinoa and chicken broth in a small saucepan and bring to a boil. Cover and lower to a simmer. Cook for about 15 minutes, or until all liquid is absorbed and quinoa is fluffy.

2. Transfer quinoa to a mixing bowl. Add cherry tomatoes, cucumber, chickpeas, kalamata olives, feta cheese, fresh mint, and fresh parsley.

3. In a separate small bowl, whisk together olive oil, lemon juice, and garlic. Pour over quinoa mixture and toss to combine.

4. Serve warm or refrigerate and serve chilled.

Recipe Tips

- Quinoa is a grain widely found in grocery stores and markets nationwide. It is usually located near the rice and other grains.
- Other varieties of beans and olives can be substituted for the chickpeas and kalamata olives if preferred.
- To hasten assembly at mealtime, make the dressing ahead and store in an airtight container in the refrigerator. Chop the vegetables earlier in the day and refrigerate.
- This is a recipe that tastes as good left over as when freshly made.

CHOICES/EXCHANGES

2 Starch, 1 Lean Protein, 1 1/2 Fat

BASIC NUTRITIONAL VALUES

Calories	270	**Potassium**	455 mg
Calories from Fat	110	**Total Carbohydrate**	32 g
Total Fat	12.0 g	Dietary Fiber	5 g
Saturated Fat	2.2 g	Sugars	5 g
Trans Fat	0.0 g	**Protein**	11 g
Cholesterol	10 mg	**Phosphorus**	255 mg
Sodium	450 mg		

Food for Thought

- **Portion sizes matter.** Portion sizes are a big concern no matter which eating pattern you embrace, because larger portions mean more calories, more carbohydrate, and thus a greater impact on blood glucose levels and weight.
- **Build awareness of portion sizes.** Check out available nutrition information. Familiarize yourself with the sizes of your dishes and glasses.
- **Use tools of the trade.** Use measuring tools, hand estimates, and comparisons of food portions to common household items to determine portion sizes and associated carbohydrate content.
- **Use smaller dishes** so portions appear larger.
- **Use preportioned foods when possible.**
- **View it before you chew it.** Put everything you eat in a dish or bowl so you can see exactly how much you're eating and make adjustments as necessary to achieve your carbohydrate targets.
- **Make swaps where you can** to save calories.
- **Embrace mindful eating** and remember the two- to three-bite taste test.

Would you consider going on a cross-country trip without a GPS, directions, or a map to guide you? Of course not! Without this important information to keep you on track, you'd soon be hopelessly lost. Even now, in your journey with type 2 diabetes, you might find yourself feeling a bit bewildered as you navigate among all the food choices available to fit into your diabetes meal plan. Fortunately, as you embrace making your own decisions about food, you have a powerful tool available to you: the nutrition information label on food and beverage packages.

What can the nutrition information on food labels do for you? It can help you ...

- Make informed food and beverage choices
- Maintain healthy eating practices

More than half of Americans say they check nutrition information labels to get a general idea of the nutrient content of their food. However, because of the overwhelming amount of label information to sift through, people often become confused, and many admit that even when the nutrition information is not healthful, they still buy the food! In this chapter, you will learn to cut through the confusion and focus on the information you need to know to successfully make the best choices for you.

Staking the Claims

The labels on foods and beverages are regulated by the United States Department of Agriculture (USDA) and the Food and Drug Administration (FDA). Most packaged foods are required by law to display nutrition labeling, although it is voluntary on raw foods such as fruits, vegetables, and fish. To learn more about foods that don't have labels, like bananas or potatoes, you may want to check out a free online database such as Calorie King (www.calorieking.com) or SuperTracker (www.supertracker.usda.gov), use a mobile app, or check out one of many guidebooks, such as *The Diabetes Carbohydrate & Fat Gram Guide, 4th Edition* by Lea Ann Holzmeister, RD, CDE, published by the American Diabetes Association.

The USDA and the FDA mandate that claims on food products must be truthful to prevent deception, examples of which include ordinary bread being touted as whole wheat or misleading claims on energy drinks.

3 Type of Claims that Manufacturers Can Make on Product Labels

#1: Health Claims

Health claims are food label messages that describe the relationship between a food component and a health-related condition (such as sodium and hypertension or calcium and osteoporosis). At the time of publication, there are a number of authorized health claims, but none related to diabetes.

Health Claim Example: "Diets low in sodium may reduce the risk of high blood pressure, a disease associated with many factors." Of course, if a food features a specific health claim, it must meet strict nutrient content requirements without being fortified. For example,

a food with a low-sodium health claim must meet the requirement for a low-sodium food (140 mg or less of sodium per serving).

#2: Nutrient Content Claims

A nutrient content claim is a word or phrase on a food package that makes a comment (directly or by implication) about the nutritional value of the food using terms such as "free, low, reduced, fewer, high, less, more, lean, extra lean, good source, or light." Nutrient content claims are strictly defined by regulations and describe the relative amount of a nutrient in a food, without specifying its exact quantity. They give a general idea about the amount of a specific nutrient in a food product. These claims generally appear on the front of food packaging. Nutrition labeling is required for virtually all nutrient content claims.

Nutrient Content Claim Example: *"Sugar free"* means the food or drink has <0.5 grams of sugar per serving. *"Reduced calorie"* means the food or drink has at least 25% fewer calories per serving than a comparable regular food or drink.

#3: Structure/Function Claims

Structure or function claims describe the role of a nutrient or dietary ingredient intended to affect the normal structure or function in humans (such as "calcium supports building strong bones"). Under the Dietary Supplement Health and Education Act (DSHEA) of 1994, structure and function claims may be used as long as such statements do not claim to diagnose, mitigate, treat, cure, or prevent disease and are not false or misleading.

Structure/Function Claim Example: "Fiber maintains bowel regularity," or "Antioxidants maintain cell integrity."

Check out the FDA website (www.fda.gov) for the most current guidelines and definitions of product label claims.

Are "Natural," "Organic," and "Healthy" Products Better For You?

If the package says a food is "natural," "organic," "vegan," "protein rich," or "kale-infused," it's got to be good for you, right? Not so fast. These buzzwords abound on grocery store shelves these days, and often cause confusion. Yes, some of these products are good for you, and some are less so. Consumers often perceive that "natural" and "organic" imply healthy! But that's not always the case. Take a closer look at the product and the nutrition information.

According to the FDA, by definition:

- **"Natural"** means the product does not contain synthetic or artificial ingredients.
- **"Organic"** foods must meet the standards set by the U.S. Department of Agriculture (USDA). Organic food differs from conventionally produced food in the way it is grown or produced. Overall, organic operations must demonstrate that they protect natural resources, use only approved

substances, and conserve biodiversity. But the USDA makes no claims that organically produced food is safer or more nutritious than conventionally produced food.
- **"Healthy"** means the product must meet certain criteria that limit the amount of fat, saturated fat, cholesterol, and sodium, and the product must contain specific minimum amounts of vitamins, minerals, or other beneficial nutrients.

Just because a food is "natural" or "organic" does not necessarily mean that it's "healthy." Some food for thought:

- Although "natural" potato chips might be made with "all-natural" ingredients, they may still be too high in carbohydrate, fat, or sodium to be "healthy" for you.
- Although a premium vanilla ice cream could be "natural" or "organic," it's still high in sugar, fat, and saturated fat, so would not meet the above criteria for "healthy."

Are "Diabetic" Foods Better for You?

When it comes to "diabetic" foods, proceed with your eyes wide open. Many sugar-free, fat-free, or reduced-fat products that are perceived as "diabetes friendly" are in fact made with ingredients that contain carbohydrate (meaning they can raise your blood glucose).

So, even if a product is touted as "sugar free" or "diabetes-friendly," you'll still want to check the label closely for the total carbohydrate content.

Case in point, revisiting ice cream again—a name-brand "low-fat, no-sugar-added" vanilla ice cream sandwich has 29 grams of carbohydrate. The regular "low-fat" version has 30 grams of carbohydrate. *Which one would you choose?* Your taste buds may tell you to go with the regular low-fat version (which generally will cost less than the "sugar-free" version too). In this case, follow your taste buds and go with the regular low-fat version over the sugar-free version.

Gluten-Free Guidance

"What is gluten?" you may wonder. Gluten is a protein in barley, rye, and wheat. Gluten is also found in crossbred hybrid grains such as triticale, which is a cross between wheat and rye. People who don't eat gluten also need to be cautious with oats; while they do not innately have gluten, they may come into contact with gluten during processing. If gluten is a concern for you do *not* eat oats unless they are labeled gluten free!

Knowing about gluten is of utmost importance for those living with celiac disease. An estimated three million people in the U.S. have celiac disease. In fact, you may have heard of the higher prevalence of celiac disease among those living with type 1 diabetes in particular.

For those with celiac disease, eating gluten triggers the production of antibodies that attack and damage the lining of the small intestine, leading to an array of uncomfortable symptoms. Such damage limits the ability of the small intestine to absorb nutrients and increases the risk for other serious health problems, including nutritional deficiencies (such as vitamin D deficiency), osteoporosis, growth retardation, infertility, miscarriages, short stature, and intestinal cancers.

The only way to manage celiac disease is to completely avoid all foods that contain gluten. Following a gluten-free lifestyle helps prevent permanent damage to the body and helps those with celiac disease feel better.

There are many people who are told they are gluten intolerant. These people also experience uncomfortable symptoms when consuming items with gluten; however, they test negative for celiac disease and actual damage to their intestine does not occur. Avoiding foods with gluten also helps relieve symptoms for those who are gluten intolerant. As for others who choose gluten-free food as a lifestyle choice, experts say there is no evidence that it's a healthier option for people not suffering from gluten intolerance or celiac disease.

If you cannot eat gluten, always read product labels carefully. Labeling standards are in place to ensure that items labeled "gluten-free" meet a standard for gluten content, thus instilling confidence that "gluten-free" items are safe for consumption.

Defining "Gluten-Free"

By definition, according to the FDA, foods labeled "gluten-free" must contain

<20 parts per million (ppm) gluten. The standard definition for "gluten-free" is as follows:

- Foods are inherently gluten-free.
- Foods must not contain an ingredient that is:
  - a gluten-containing grain (such as spelt wheat);
  - derived from a gluten-containing grain that has not been processed to remove gluten (such as wheat flour); OR
  - derived from a gluten-containing grain that has been processed to remove gluten (such as wheat starch), if the use of that ingredient results in the presence of 20 ppm or more gluten in the food.

Restaurants and other establishments making a gluten-free claim on their menus should be consistent with the FDA's definition.

If celiac disease or gluten intolerance is a concern for you, talk with your registered dietitian/registered dietitian nutritionist (RD/RDN) or doctor for further guidance on gluten-free eating.

What Do You *Really* Need to Know to Make Good Food Choices?

If you've occasionally (or maybe frequently) taken a look at nutrition information labels over the years, you've probably noticed that a lot has changed since these labels made their debut over 20 years ago! Although it may be interesting and nice to see health claims and the exact details for each nutrient on a label, you don't have to memorize the FDA/USDA regulations to make the best choices for your diabetes meal plan!

If you find yourself standing in the supermarket aisle trying to decide which loaf of bread to buy, at first glance, the information on the label may seem overwhelming. Rather than throwing your hands up in frustration and randomly choosing a bread to toss in your shopping basket, take another moment to check out the label. What you really need to know is how to compare the nutrient numbers and claims of the different breads.

To provide a point of reference and get you started on your quest to make good-for-you choices, **there are some quick tips in Table 4.1 about the nutrients on nutrition information labels** that have the most impact on your diabetes.

Ultimately, the goal is to build awareness of what you eat and become empowered to make the choices that are best for you. After all, not all healthful-sounding products are created equal.

Top 10 Label Features That Deserve Your Attention

At the time this book was published, FDA food labeling regulations were in flux and the nutrition information label format was in the

Table 4.1	Nutrient Quick Tips
Nutrient	**Quick tip**
Calories	Guide to calories in a single serving of a food: • 40 calories is low • 100 calories is moderate • 400 or more calories is high
Fats	Limit your intake of: • Saturated fat • Trans fat • Cholesterol
Sodium	The percent daily value of sodium, at time of publication, is based on 2,400 mg/day. This is similar to the recommendation for people with diabetes, which is 2,300 mg/day or less.
Total carbohydrates Dietary fiber Sugars Sugar alcohols (Polyols)	Don't just focus on grams of sugar. Total carbohydrate is what affects your blood glucose most directly. The grams of total carbohydrate listed on nutrition information labels already include starch, fiber, sugars, and sugar alcohols—you don't have to add those to total carbohydrate.
	If you're counting carbohydrate choices (servings), approximately 15 grams of total carbohydrate = 1 carbohydrate choice (serving).
	Foods containing >3 grams of dietary fiber per serving are considered *high in fiber,* according to the Academy of Nutrition and Dietetics and American Diabetes Association's booklet *Choose Your Foods: Food Lists for Diabetes.* A high-fiber food that has at least 5 grams of dietary fiber per serving is considered an *excellent source* of fiber.
	Dietary fiber and sugar alcohols can influence the way carbohydrate affects your blood glucose and may need special consideration (see Chapter 2 for more information).

process of being redesigned. But regardless of how the final refreshed label design, its content, or labeling regulations turn out, there are 10 core pieces of information—or "features"—on the nutrition information label that you can use to make the best food choices for you:

Feature #1: Ingredient List

First things first: Peruse the ingredient list to check out what is in your food or beverage. When you look at the list of ingredients on a label, remember that they are listed in descending order by weight. This means that the first ingredient is the main (heaviest) ingredient, followed by ingredients used in lesser amounts.

Take, for example, the following ingredient lists from two different steam-in-the-bag broccoli products:

- Frozen steam-in-the-bag broccoli florets have one ingredient: broccoli.
- Frozen steam-in-the-bag broccoli with cheese sauce contains broccoli *plus* nearly 20 other ingredients.

Also pay attention to whether the food product has healthier ingredients (such as whole-wheat flour or canola oil) or not-so-healthy ingredients (such as hydrogenated or partially hydrogenated oils).

Takeaway: Know what you're eating. If you don't recognize multiple ingredients in the item, maybe it's best put back on the shelf. You can make healthier choices just by choosing items that have healthier ingredients listed first in the ingredient list.

Feature #2: Serving Size and Servings Per Container

Size up the serving size and the number of servings in the package/container. The serving size on a food or beverage label is a standardized amount used for comparing similar foods/beverages. It may be different from the portion you usually eat/drink or the serving sizes in your meal plan. As you learned in Chapter 3, portion size matters! Once you've determined the serving size of a food, you're on the way to knowing the exact amounts of nutrients you'll be getting from that food.

Let's use popcorn as an example. If you pop up some light microwave popcorn, do you eat a 3-cup serving? Or the 6.5-cup serving listed on the bag? Or the entire bag?

Take a look at the selected nutrition information below, which is from a box of light microwave popcorn:

- Serving size: about 6.5 cups popped
- Servings per bag: about 2
- Calories per serving: 120
- Total carbohydrate: 25 grams

Takeaway: As you can see, the serving size for this light microwave popcorn is 6.5 cups popped, which has 120 calories and 25 grams of carbohydrate. However, the number of servings per container is two. So, if you eat the entire bag of popcorn (even though it is "light"), you'll be munching down 50 grams of carbohydrate—nearly enough carbohydrate for a meal! That extra carbohydrate can make quite a difference in your blood glucose, particularly if excess consumption like this happens several times a day!

Food Lists

If you use the Academy of Nutrition and Dietetics/American Diabetes Association booklet *Choose Your Foods: Food Lists for Diabetes* for meal planning purposes, remember that each food list groups foods together because they have similar nutrient content and serving sizes. Each serving on a food list has about the same amount of calories, carbohydrate, protein, and fat as the other foods on that same list. Be prepared to do a little math to translate the serving size on the label to the serving size called for in your meal plan. There are many mobile apps and free, online food databases that enable you to adjust the serving size of the food of interest in order to see the associated nutrient content information. Or you can pull out a good old calculator or smartphone calculator to get the job done.

Again, at the time this book was published, the FDA was in the process of redesigning and updating nutrition information labels. Serving sizes—one of the label features undergoing change—are predicted to begin to look more realistic; they will be based on the portions people usually consume in one sitting, rather than what they "should" be eating.

Feature #3: Percent Daily Value

What is Percent Daily Value?

The percent daily value (% DV) information on the label may initially bring some confusion. The *Dietary Guidelines for Americans* (www.health.gov/dietaryguidelines) recommends specific amounts of certain nutrients each day for optimum health. While nutrition and calorie needs may vary from person to person, the % DV on food and beverage packages are based on an average 2,000-calorie-per-day meal plan to provide a point of comparison.

Take a Closer Look: Food List Serving Sizes

Food	Label serving size	Food list serving size
Almonds	28 nuts (1 ounce)	6 nuts
English muffin	1 muffin	1/2 muffin
Raisins	1/4 cup	2 tablespoons
Brown rice	2/3 cup cooked	1/3 cup cooked

Serving sizes are based on Academy of Nutrition and Dietetics and American Diabetes Association. Choose Your Foods: Food Lists for Diabetes. *Washington, DC, Academy of Nutrition and Dietetics, American Diabetes Association, 2014*

What Does % DV Mean for You?

1. Glancing at % DV can help you see what and how much you're getting from what you're eating in the context of average needs for a day. These values can help you understand whether a food/beverage contributes a little or a lot of a particular nutrient to your total daily diet.

    A quick guide to % DV: 5% or less is low, 20% or more is high.

    Take sodium, for example:
    - 5% DV (120 mg) or less of sodium per serving is low
    - 20% DV (480 mg) or more of sodium per serving is high

2. Percent daily value can help you to track and raise or lower your intake of particular nutrients as needed.

    Your meal plan might not be based on 2,000 calories per day, but the % DV is still a good frame of reference. At your next visit with your RD/RDN or certified diabetes educator, you may want to take a few minutes to calculate your own personal daily values for key nutrients and keep those numbers handy. You'll then be able to judge how far the amount of fat or fiber, for example, in a food goes toward meeting your individual nutrition goals.

    Take fiber and vitamin D, for instance:

    Let's say on the nutrition information label for a food, the amount of dietary fiber is 35% DV, which makes this food an excellent source of fiber; however, if vitamin D is 0% DV, this item is not a good source of vitamin D. You might decide to either eat or forgo this food based on how much of these particular nutrients you need.

3. You can also use % DV to compare similar foods and determine which is best for you.

For example, what if you're trying to eat heart-healthy and reduce your saturated fat, trans fat, and cholesterol intake, but you love a little cheese now and then? Let's compare the % DV of these nutrients in two kinds of cheese to determine which will better meet your nutrition goal.

	Cheddar cheese	Light cheddar cheese
Saturated fat	6 g (30% DV)	3 g (16% DV)
Trans fat	0 g	0 g
Cholesterol	30 mg (10% DV)	15 mg (5% DV)

Takeaway: Between the two cheeses, the light cheddar would be the better choice because the % DV for saturated fat and cholesterol are lower than those for the regular cheddar cheese.

Some nutrients, such as trans fat, sugars, and protein, don't have a % DV listing. This is because no daily reference value has been established for these nutrients. However, you can still use the amount per serving to make comparisons between products before you buy.

> ## Trans Fat Tips
>
> If a serving of a food contains <0.5 grams of trans fat, it may be noted on the label as containing "0 grams" of trans fat. But several servings of a food that contains 0.4 grams of trans fat, while technically labeled as having "0 grams" of trans fat per serving, can add up! There is no % DV for trans fat, but you should keep your consumption as low as possible, preferably avoiding trans fat altogether.

Feature #4: Calories

While you may hone your focus in on carbohydrate to help achieve blood glucose control, calories do still matter. The number of calories per serving is especially important to maintain a healthy weight. (See Chapter 1 for additional guidance.) **Look at the number of calories per serving on each food.** How many of those servings do you plan to eat? Two? If you double the serving, then double the calories.

Checking out calories can provide perspective in the context of your daily calorie goal.

Take pistachios, for instance:

1/2 cup pistachios equals 350 calories. If you're trying to lose weight and hold your calories around 1,500 per day, that 1/2 cup of nuts uses up nearly one-quarter of your day's calories!

Are There "Free" Foods?

A serving of a food/beverage with <20 calories and <5 grams of carbohydrate may be counted as a "free" food. Limit yourself to three servings or fewer of the "free" food per day and spread these servings out throughout the day; otherwise, the carbohydrate in the item may raise your blood glucose. So "free" doesn't mean "unlimited free."

Consider salsa:

Want to use 1/4 cup fresh salsa to top grilled chicken? A 1/4-cup portion of salsa is a "free" food. However, if you want to use 1 cup of salsa to slather over a bean burrito, the larger portion of salsa is *not* "free" and must be counted.

Feature #5: Fat

As we'll discuss later in Chapter 8, the *type* of fat eaten is more important than the *total amount* of fat. With the goal in mind to choose foods that are limited in saturated fat and cholesterol with zero trans fat, and those that are rich in heart-healthy polyunsaturated and monounsaturated fat, turn to the nutrition information label. The label shares with you the amounts of the following fats in the item:

- Total fat
- Saturated fat
- Trans fat
- Polyunsaturated fat
- Monounsaturated fat

	Mayonnaise	Extra-virgin olive oil mayonnaise	Guacamole
Serving size	1 tablespoon	1 tablespoon	1 tablespoon
Total fat	10 g	5 g	3 g
Saturated fat	1.5 g	0.5 g	0 g
Trans fat	0 g	0 g	0 g
Cholesterol	5 mg	5 mg	0 mg

Let's take a look at real mayonnaise—a food in which nearly all of the calories come from fat—in comparison to a couple of other creamy sandwich spread options. When it comes to fat, by comparison, which of these spreads would you choose?

Takeaway: Choose guacamole for the healthiest fat profile, followed by the mayo made with extra-virgin olive oil (as opposed to regular mayo).

Feature #6: Total Carbohydrate

When it comes to carbohydrate, know your numbers. (See Chapters 1 and 2 for detailed guidance related to carbohydrate.) Check the grams of "Total Carbohydrate" per serving on the nutrition information label. The number of total carbohydrate *does* include the grams of dietary fiber and sugars, so you do not need to count those separately or add them to the Total Carbohydrate. Total carbohydrate is "one-stop shopping" when it comes to counting carbohydrates; that's the number to use in your carbohydrate count. (As an aside, take care NOT to interpret the gram weight of the serving—as denoted alongside the serving size on the label—as the grams of carbohydrate. We've found in practice over the years that some of our patients confuse the two.)

Compare total carbohydrate amounts among items to see what best fits your nutrition needs. **We compare two types of cereal—bran flake cereal and frosted flake cereal—below to see how this works.**

Takeaway: The carbohydrate content of these two flake cereals is close, although the Total Carbohydrate in the bran flake cereal is 3 grams less than that of the frosted flake cereal.

	Bran flake cereal	Frosted flake cereal
Serving size	1 cup	1 cup
Total carbohydrate	32 g	35 g
Dietary fiber	7 g	0.7 g

And the fiber of the bran flakes is 10 times more! That's a big plus! *Which would you choose?*

Feature #7: Added Sugars

While the total carbohydrate count (See "Feature #6") is your overarching focus for blood glucose control, the "Added Sugars" information is particularly eye-opening. The goal of this information is to help you distinguish between sugars that are naturally found in foods/beverages (such as those in fruit/natural fruit juice) and the refined sugars added by food manufacturers. On average Americans get 16% of their daily calories from sugars added during food production. That's too much. Foods and beverages with added sugars can decrease your intake of nutrient-rich foods while increasing calorie intake. Furthermore, there's solid evidence linking excessive sugar consumption to an increased risk for heart disease and other illnesses.

The grams of added sugar are encompassed in the "Total Carbohydrate" value on nutrition information labels, so they do not need to be accounted for separately in terms of carbohydrate count. However, added sugars provide no added nutrition, and thus are often referred to as "empty calories."

You can easily spot added sugars as you peruse the ingredient list. **Words that mean "added sugar" include the following:**

- Added sugars (brown, cane, confectioner's, date, invert, powdered, turbinado)
- Agave nectar
- Dextrose
- Fructose

- Honey
- Maltose
- Molasses
- Polydextrose
- Sucrose
- Syrup (corn, maple, agave)

Every 4 grams of sugar is equal to 1 teaspoon of sugar! Choose items without added sugars among the first three ingredients. Compare brands of similar products and choose those with the least amount of added sugars.

Take canned sliced peaches as an example:

Peaches canned in 100% juice have no added sugars, while those canned in heavy syrup generally have two or more types of added sugars, resulting in a total carbohydrate count over 1 1/2 times that of the peaches without added sugar!

Takeaway: To conserve carbohydrate and consume less added sugar, choose fruit canned in juice over that canned in syrup.

Your palate may benefit from less sugar as you begin to appreciate the natural sweetness of many foods. (See Chapters 2 and 8 for additional guidance on added sweeteners.)

Feature #8: Fiber

When reading nutrition information labels, look for foods rich in "Dietary Fiber." Foods containing >3 grams of dietary fiber per serving are considered "high in fiber," according to the Academy of Nutrition and Dietetics and American Diabetes Association booklet *Choose Your Foods: Food Lists for Diabetes.* A high-fiber food that has at least 5 grams of dietary fiber per serving is considered an excellent source of fiber. (See Chapter 8 for additional detailed guidance on fiber.)

Compare the fiber amounts in these soups, for example:

- 1 cup chicken noodle soup = 0.7 g fiber
- 1 cup black bean soup = 8 g fiber

Takeaway: The black bean soup has over 11 times the fiber of chicken noodle soup and is considered an excellent source of fiber.

Look again at the earlier cereal comparison in "Feature #6: Total Carbohydrate" (page 73) and check out the difference in fiber between bran flake cereal and frosted flake cereal.

Takeaway: The fiber in bran flakes is 10 times that in frosted flakes! So bran flakes would be a much better cereal choice.

Feature #9: Sodium and Potassium

Give sodium and potassium a little extra attention if you're concerned about high blood pressure. Eating less sodium can help manage blood pressure. And eating more potassium-rich foods may help lower blood pressure and prevent high blood pressure. In general, Americans don't consume enough potassium. (See Chapter 8 for additional specific guidance.)

When reading a nutrition information label, check out the "Sodium" value and see how the food fits within your daily sodium limits. And choose foods that are high in potassium (unless your health-care team advises you otherwise).

Check out the sodium content in tomatoes, which are rich in potassium, for example:

- 1/2 cup diced fresh = only 5 mg sodium
- 1/2 cup diced canned = 130 mg sodium

Takeaway: To get a potassium boost but manage sodium, go for diced fresh tomatoes instead of diced canned tomatoes (or choose no-salt-added canned tomatoes).

Feature #10: Vitamin D

In general, Americans don't consume enough vitamin D, which is important for healthy, strong bones, especially for women and older adults. Look for foods and beverages that are rich in vitamin D to get the most nutrition for your calories. At the time this book was published, vitamin D was not listed on nutrition information labels, but it is one of the FDA's proposed additions to the forthcoming label design. Remember 20% daily value or more is a high percent daily value.

Take the Time to Read Labels

Reading labels can add some time to your grocery shopping routine (at least initially), so you may want to set aside a few moments to study the labels on the foods you often purchase. Compare the labels of your choices side by side. Once you've identified the best choices for your grocery staples, your future shopping trips will go much faster. Even after you've identified your favorites, periodically do a checkup on their labels to catch any changes in ingredients and numbers. The time you spend now will save you time—and protect your health—for years into the future.

Take One Last Look at the Label

Limit these nutrients	Get enough of these nutrients
Saturated Fat	Dietary Fiber
Trans Fat	Potassium
Cholesterol	
Sodium	
Added Sugars	

Make a Smart Choice: It's All About You!

You've taken a good look at a nutrition information label to size up your servings and learn more about the specific nutrients in each serving. Now it's time for you to make a smart choice, keeping your own personal needs and diabetes care in mind. **Here are two additional special tips on label reading:**

Tip #1: "Sugar Free" Isn't "Carbohydrate Free"

Technically, if a food is labeled "sugar free," it has <0.5 grams of sugar per serving. However, sugar-free foods may still contain carbohydrate, especially if sweeteners such as sugar alcohols (also known as polyols) are used in their preparation. (See Chapter 2 for more information about sugar alcohols.) Sugar alcohols may be listed on the nutrition information label. As a reminder, sugar alcohols do contain calories and carbohydrate, which can boost your blood glucose levels, particularly if you eat a large serving

of them. Check your blood glucose after eating them to note their effect on you.

Candy Comparison

Comparing the nutrition information labels of a standard product and its sugar-free version you may be surprised to find that there is little difference in the carbohydrate content. Or, that the sugar-free variety is actually higher in carbohydrate than the standard version, as is the scenario with the butterscotch hard candy below. If that is the case, let your taste and your budget guide your choice.

Butterscotch hard candy	Carbohydrate (grams)
1 piece regular	4.8
1 piece sugar free	5.7

Tip #2: Fat-Free Foods Often Contain Carbs

If you're counting calories, fat-free foods may seem like a great solution to a dieting dilemma. However, many of today's fat replacers are carbohydrate based. Although the fat content in a product might be lower, the carbohydrate content can be higher and affect your blood glucose. You'll find an example on the following page.

Takeaway: After reading the nutrition information label and finding that the fat-free version of ranch salad dressing contains a significant amount of carbohydrate, you may decide to eat a small portion of the "real thing."

Food	Calories	Fat (grams)	Carbohydrate (grams)
2 tablespoons regular ranch salad dressing	140	14	2
2 tablespoons fat-free ranch salad dressing	30	0	6

Next Steps

Put your label-reading skills to the test by doing a bit of shelf searching. Find three foods in your pantry that fall into each of the following categories:

- Contains 0–15 grams of carbohydrate per serving
- Contains 16–30 grams of carbohydrate per serving
- Contains 31–45 grams of carbohydrate per serving

Did you note the serving size and number of servings per package on the foods you found?

What Do I Eat for Breakfast?

FOR 45–60 GRAMS OF CARBOHYDRATE*
Recipe: Lean Green Smoothie or Cherry
  Berry Smoothie (3/4 cup)
1 scrambled egg or 1/4 cup egg substitute
2 slices whole-grain toast with 2 teaspoons
  honey

FOR 60–75 GRAMS OF CARBOHYDRATE*
Recipe: Lean Green Smoothie or Cherry
  Berry Smoothie (3/4 cup)
1 scrambled egg or 1/4 cup egg substitute
2 slices whole-grain toast with 2 teaspoons honey
1/2 cup cooked oatmeal or cream of wheat
  with cinnamon

*For most women, 45–60 grams of carbohydrate at a meal is a good starting point; for most men, 60–75 grams of carbohydrate per meal is appropriate. Check with your diabetes health-care team to find the amount of carbohydrate that's right for you.

Swift, Simple Tips

- Whip up the smoothies while the toast is toasting and the egg is cooking.
- Consider making a double portion of oatmeal or cream of wheat and refrigerating the second portion in a mug to heat up the following morning. Thin with water or low-fat milk.
- Both smoothies can also easily stand alone as a 1–carbohydrate choice snack.

LEAN GREEN SMOOTHIE

SERVES: 4

SERVING SIZE: 3/4 cup

PREPARATION TIME: 5 minutes

COOKING TIME: 0 minutes

INGREDIENTS

1 cup unsweetened vanilla-flavored
   almond milk

2 cups raw baby spinach

1 cup fat-free plain greek yogurt

1 cup unsweetened frozen diced pineapple

3 large ice cubes

4 dashes ground cinnamon

1. Combine almond milk, spinach, yogurt, pineapple, and ice in a blender. Cover and blend until smooth. Pour into 4 glasses and garnish each serving with a dash of ground cinnamon. Serve immediately.

A Bit about Almond Milk

Unsweetened vanilla-flavored almond milk is made from finely ground almonds and water. It generally has fewer calories than cow's milk and contains no cholesterol, trans fat, or saturated fat. The amount of carbohydrate in almond milk depends on the brand you buy, and the unsweetened variety may contain as little as 1 gram of carbohydrate per serving. Almond milk is often fortified with vitamins and minerals, but read the label before you buy for more specific information. Although almond milk is nutritious and contains a variety of essential nutrients, it's not a good source of protein, containing only 1 gram of protein per cup versus 8 grams of protein in a cup of cow's milk.

CHOICES/EXCHANGES

1/2 Carbohydrate,
1 Lean Protein

BASIC NUTRITIONAL VALUES

Calories	70	**Potassium**	330 mg
Calories from Fat	10	**Total Carbohydrate**	9 g
Total Fat	1.0 g	Dietary Fiber	1 g
Saturated Fat	0.1 g	Sugars	7 g
Trans Fat	0.0 g	**Protein**	7 g
Cholesterol	0 mg	**Phosphorus**	100 mg
Sodium	90 mg		

CHERRY BERRY SMOOTHIE

SERVES: 4

SERVING SIZE: 3/4 cup

PREPARATION TIME: 5 minutes

COOKING TIME: 0 minutes

INGREDIENTS

1 1/2 cups unsweetened pitted frozen
  dark sweet or sour cherries

1 cup unsweetened vanilla-flavored
  almond milk

1 (6-ounce) carton fat-free blueberry-flavored
  greek yogurt

1/2 cup fresh or frozen unsweetened
  blueberries

1 small banana, peeled and chopped into
  large pieces

1. Combine cherries, almond milk, yogurt, blueberries, and banana in a blender. Cover and blend until smooth. Pour into glasses and serve immediately.

Recipe Tips

- Not only is using frozen fruit in a smoothie often less expensive than using fresh, it also gives the smoothie a frosty, creamy texture without the need for adding ice and diluting the flavor of your drink.
- Buy prewashed, bagged baby spinach for the Lean Green Smoothie.
- If you plan ahead, you can also freeze the peeled and chopped banana before using it in the Cherry Berry Smoothie. In fact, we often toss overly ripe unpeeled bananas in the freezer, then thaw slightly, peel, and use in smoothies such as this one.

CHOICES/EXCHANGES
1 Fruit, 1 Lean Protein

BASIC NUTRITIONAL VALUES

Calories	90	**Potassium**	265 mg
Calories from Fat	15	**Total Carbohydrate**	18 g
Total Fat	1.5 g	Dietary Fiber	2 g
Saturated Fat	0.2 g	Sugars	12 g
Trans Fat	0.0 g	**Protein**	5 g
Cholesterol	5 mg	**Phosphorus**	65 mg
Sodium	60 mg		

Food for Thought

- **Size up your servings.**
- **Know your numbers.** Check the out the labels of the foods you eat, paying special attention to the numbers for the 10 features outlined in this chapter.
- **Make smart food choices**—it's all about you.
- Feel overwhelmed by the nutrition information label? Get back to basics and focus on serving size and amount of total carbohydrate.

As you've learned in the previous chapters, what you eat plays a major role in keeping you healthy, strong, and in control of your diabetes. Remember what we pointed out earlier in this book: following every one of the medical recommendations for diabetes self-care would take at least 143 minutes of your day. Of that time, 57 minutes are related to food—meal planning, grocery shopping, and preparing meals! Although you may already know exactly what you're supposed to eat, you'll still need to take several steps to make the transition from *knowing* what you need to do to actually sitting down and enjoying a great-tasting, healthy meal. Unless you have a personal dietitian, shopper, and chef, you'll be the one responsible for planning menus, shopping for food, and preparing meals to meet your diabetes needs. This chapter is designed to help you get the most out of those 57 minutes by focusing on smarter planning, smarter shopping, and smarter cooking!

Plan Smart

Winston Churchill once said, "Let our advance worrying become advance thinking and planning." Are you feeling anxious about when, where, and what you should be eating? You can change that anxiety into action by planning your meals and snacks in advance. Listen to Sarah, a busy accountant with type 2 diabetes:

> *"I've found that if I spend a little time thinking about and preparing food for the week ahead, I make better choices at meals and snack time. If I haven't thought things through, I find myself heading for the nearest*

fast-food drive-thru on my way home from work. But if I've got a menu worked out and what I need to prepare a quick and healthy dinner in my kitchen at home, I make much better food choices. Taking a few moments to plan my meals and snacks makes me healthier and often saves me money, too."

Both Winston Churchill and Sarah have pointed out some of the important reasons for you to plan your meals in advance:

- **Healthier food choices**—Taking the time to plan meals in advance lets you make sure they are balanced and meet your diabetes needs.
- **Time savings**—A five-minute upfront investment of your time will yield much bigger time savings because planning enables you to grocery shop efficiently and helps you avoid extra trips to the store for missing items.
- **Money savings**—Planning your meals ahead of time lets you create a grocery list, which translates into saving money at the checkout lane. Because you buy only what you need, in the proper package sizes, you waste less food. Eating at home, rather than paying for meals at restaurants, puts even more pennies in your piggy bank.
- **Energy savings**—Planning meals in advance not only saves our environment (by limiting those extra trips

to the grocery store), but it also saves mental energy because you don't have to sweat over what you're eating for supper. Cooking is more enjoyable when you are prepared.

Menu Planning: Where to Begin?

There's no mystery to designing a menu. All "menu planning" really means is that you decide what you'll be eating ahead of time. **Here are a few tips to help you:**

- **Know your meal plan:** You may need to schedule a visit with a registered dietitian/registered dietitian nutritionist (RD/RDN), who can review your health and nutrition history, medications, blood glucose levels, and lifestyle and then design an individualized plan that works for you. Several different diabetes meal-planning approaches are in use today (see Table 5.1 on page 84). In Chapter 1 we reviewed some eating patterns, including Mediterranean-style, vegetarian and vegan, low-fat, and low-carbohydrate eating patterns, and the DASH diet. Your choice of which eating pattern to follow is based on your personal preferences and diabetes goals. Once you know the number of servings you need each day from each food group, you have the outline of your basic meal plan. That outline then translates into your menu, which then becomes your shopping list.

Planned Overs

"The most remarkable thing about my mother is that for 30 years she served the family nothing but leftovers. The original meal has never been found."—Calvin Trillin

No one wants to eat the same meal day after day, but "planned overs" are a smart cook's best friend. Planned overs are key ingredients you have deliberately saved after a meal to use as part of another meal later on. In other words, you're planning ahead by making more of an ingredient than you'll eat in one meal! Here are some examples of how you can use leftover ingredients:

- After serving a roasted turkey breast, use the extra meat the next day in a turkey pot pie.
- Make a stir-fry using extra chunks of cooked chicken breast along with fresh oriental vegetables and brown rice.
- Transform the extra pork from a pork roast into a zesty chili with kidney beans, tomatoes, zucchini, and your favorite spices.

Design your menus with an eye for planned overs to save time and money!

- **Plan a week in advance:** Don't overwhelm yourself by creating menus more than a week in advance. Get started with dinner. Pull out your calendar, and note what you'll be doing each evening during the upcoming week. Perhaps a business dinner or children's activity means you'll be eating away from home, so that's one less dinner to plan.
- **Rely on favorites:** Go through your recipe box, files, cookbooks, and other

It Takes Just 5 Steps to Plan 5 Meals

1. Divide a piece of paper into three columns.
2. In one column, list five or more of your/your family's favorite main dish items.
3. In the second column, list several vegetables and fruits you/your family consistently enjoy(s).
4. In the third column, list the types of grains you/your family enjoy(s).
5. Mix and match the items in each column to plan five meals.

favorite sources, and pick out several recipes that are tried and true. Note how they fit into your diabetes meal plan. (See Chapter 9 if you need to learn about improving the nutrition

value of some of your favorite recipes.) These recipes will be the heart of your meal plan. The recipes in this book are also created to spark your meal-planning creativity.

Table 5.1	Meal-Planning Approaches	
Meal-planning approach	**Quick overview**	**Where can you learn more?**
Choose My Plate	Although not specifically designed for diabetes, this meal-planning approach from the USDA gives you a framework to help you make healthy food choices and be active every day. You'll be guided to select servings from each food group: fruits, vegetables, grains, protein foods, dairy, and oils.	**U.S. Department of Agriculture (USDA)** www.ChooseMyPlate.gov
Create Your Plate	This step-by-step guide to filling your plate shows the proper portion sizes and number of servings you need to eat from each food group: nonstarchy vegetables, grains and starchy foods, protein, fruit, and dairy. Your RD/RDN will help individualize this plan for you.	**American Diabetes Association** www.diabetes.org
Choose Your Foods: Food Lists for Diabetes	In this resource, foods are grouped together in lists with similar nutrient content and serving sizes. You and your RD/RDN will decide how many servings to select from each food group: starch, fruits, milk and milk substitutes, nonstarchy vegetables, sweets, desserts, and other carbohydrates, proteins, fats, and alcohol.	**Academy of Nutrition and Dietetics** www.eatright.org **American Diabetes Association** www.diabetes.org

Table 5.1	Meal-Planning Approaches *(Continued)*	
Meal-planning approach	**Quick overview**	**Where can you learn more?**
Carbohydrate Counting	Because carbohydrate (starch and sugar) is the main nutrient in food that raises blood glucose, this approach only counts the foods that contain carbohydrate. You'll count either the grams of carbohydrate or the carbohydrate choices/servings (1 carbohydrate choice/serving = 15 grams of carbohydrate). Your RD/RDN can help you decide how much carbohydrate you need based on your age, weight, activity, and diabetes medications.	**American Diabetes Association** www.diabetes.org American Diabetes Association Publications: • *Count Your Carbs: Getting Started* • *Match Your Insulin to Your Carbs* • *The Diabetes Carbohydrate & Fat Gram Guide, 4th Edition* • *The Complete Guide to Carb Counting, 3rd Edition*

This is not an all-inclusive list of diabetes meal-planning approaches. Check with your RD/RDN to find the plan that works best for you.

3 Little Words

To improve your menus, consider these three things:

- **Color.** More color on your plate generally means more variety and better nutrition. Skip the bland white vegetables and nondescript starches in favor of colorful green, yellow, and red vegetables, along with rich whole grains.
- **Temperature.** Vary the temperatures of your food choices at a meal—some cold foods, some at room temperature, and some hot—to add more interest.
- **Texture.** Consider crisp, crunchy, smooth, chunky, and tender foods for your menu. Including different textures automatically helps you include items from all food groups.

Shop Smart

Diabetes is an expensive condition. People with diabetes, on average, have medical costs that are about 2.3 times higher than the costs of people without diabetes. Because your budget must stretch to cover medications, monitoring supplies, and trips to the doctor, it's important for you to save money by shopping smart.

It's a common misconception that healthy foods are more expensive. Eating healthfully does require a small investment of time for planning, shopping, and cooking. However, there is no better investment in your health than good nutrition. Time and time again, research has shown that improving blood glucose control lowers the risk of diabetes complications, such as eye and kidney disease. Nutrition is a key factor in diabetes control and, contrary to popular belief, healthful eating for diabetes does not require special diabetic foods and high-priced sugar-free treats. Your nutrition plan is the same as the nutrition plan for anyone interested in eating right. It should consist of high-fiber grains, beans, fruits, and vegetables; have small portions of meat and protein foods; and include only limited amounts of fats, sweets, and alcohol.

3 Secrets of Savvy Shoppers

Let these three secrets of savvy shoppers guide you as you're learning to shop smart:

1. **Smart shoppers search for bargains in more than one type of store.**
   - Visit the warehouse club once a month to stock up on nonperishable staples in large sizes, the supercenter for low everyday prices, and the regular supermarket when you need to save time.
   - Check your local food co-op for near-wholesale prices on beans, grains, and other bulk foods.
   - Some grocery stores now have in-store nutritionists who can give you advice on making better choices in the supermarket to meet your lifestyle needs.

2. **Smart shoppers know that minimizing the number of minutes spent in the grocery store means saving money.**
   - Food marketing research has found that shoppers pay almost $2 for every minute spent inside the grocery store, meaning you should minimize your shopping time.

Cost-Friendly Recipes and Food Plans

The USDA has developed recipes and food plans designed to feed a family of four at home starting at about $150 per week (in early 2015). Visit the "USDA Food Plans: Cost of Food" page on the USDA website (www.cnpp.usda.gov) for more information.

- The first step to reducing shopping minutes in the store is to plan your menus in advance. Then make a grocery list to guide you. You'll save even more time by organizing your list to match the aisle-by-aisle layout of your grocery store. That way you won't add time to your shopping trip by doubling back to pick up forgotten items.

3. **Smart shoppers take advantage of specials, coupons, and store brands.**
   - Most grocery stores have predictable sales cycles; for example, perhaps ground beef or certain canned goods are on sale every six weeks. Make a note of these sales dates, then stock up and plan your menus around them.
   - Using coupons and store rewards programs saves you money if you use them on items you normally buy. For extra motivation, note the amount you save each week and stash that cash in a piggy bank to treat yourself to a movie or massage in the future.
   - Store brands or generic versions of products can be as much as 30% below the price of name brands. And because they are often produced by brand-name manufacturers, their quality can be quite good.

Should You Skip the Special "Diabetic" Food?

Take a moment to carefully compare the nutrition and price information for the treats below. Then decide which of these products is the smarter choice.

- One serving (five pieces) of sugar alcohol–sweetened peanut butter cup candy costs about $1.20.
- One serving (five pieces) of regular peanut butter cup candy costs about $ 0.39.

Both have about the same amount of carbohydrate and while the sugar alcohol–sweetened candy has fewer calories, it costs three times as much!

6 Smart Shopping Selections—Save $10!

Grocery store item	Smart shopping selections
Preshredded carrots 1 ounce = $0.22	Whole carrots shredded at home 1 ounce = $0.02
Marinated pork tenderloin 1 pound = $6.56	Plain pork tenderloin with spices/oil added at home 1 pound = $3.47
Brand-name toasted oat cereal 3/4 cup = $0.33	Store-brand, bagged toasted oat cereal 3/4 cup = $0.11
100-calorie snack pack of almonds 1 ounce = $0.75	Bulk packed almonds 1 ounce = $0.43
Strawberry greek yogurt 6 ounces = $1.44	Plain greek yogurt with added fresh berries 6 ounces = $0.99
Brand-name olive oil 25.5 ounces = $11.49	Store-brand olive oil 25.5 ounces = $5.69
TOTAL $20.79	TOTAL $10.71

You Save $10.08!!!

The Well-Stocked Pantry

Healthy eating is even easier if you keep a variety of basic foods on hand to make quick and healthy meals and snacks. Then you can add fresh ingredients as needed. Below are lists of several staple foods and ingredients (and cooking tools) you may want to keep in your kitchen. Many of these foods come in low-fat, low-sodium, or sugar-free versions. Choose which foods/versions to purchase based on your diabetes nutrition goals.

Canned and Packaged Goods

- Applesauce (unsweetened)
- Beans, canned and dried
- Bran
- Bread crumbs
- Broth (low sodium)
- Chicken, canned
- Fruit, dried and canned (unsweetened or packed in juice)
- Lentils
- Nuts
- Oats
- Olives, canned
- Pasta
- Pasta sauce
- Pickles
- Salmon, canned
- Soup (low sodium)
- Tomato paste
- Tomato sauce
- Tomatoes, canned
- Tuna, canned
- Vegetables, canned

Condiments

- 100% fruit preserves or reduced-sugar fruit spreads
- Barbecue sauce
- Horseradish
- Hot sauce
- Ketchup
- Lemon juice
- Mayonnaise (light)
- Mustard
- Peanut butter
- Relish
- Salad dressing
- Salsa
- Soy sauce (low sodium)
- Syrup (sugar free)
- Vinegar
- Worcestershire sauce

Cooking Staples

- Baking powder
- Baking soda
- Bouillon cubes (low sodium)
- Cocoa
- Cooking spray
- Cornmeal
- Cornstarch
- Evaporated milk
- Extracts
- Flour
- Oil (olive and/or canola)
- Powdered milk
- Sugar
- Sweeteners

(continued on next page)

The Well-Stocked Pantry *(Continued)*

Herbs and Spices

- Allspice
- Basil
- Cayenne pepper
- Chili powder
- Cinnamon
- Cloves
- Coriander (cilantro)
- Cumin
- Curry powder

- Dill
- Garlic
- Ginger
- Marjoram
- Mint
- Nutmeg
- Onion powder
- Paprika
- Parsley

- Pepper
- Red pepper flakes
- Rosemary
- Sage
- Salt
- Tarragon
- Thyme

Tools of the Trade

Having the right kitchen tools at your fingertips makes cooking easier and more enjoyable. Here are some common kitchen tools you may want to have handy:

- Baking dishes, glass
- Baking sheets
- Blender
- Cheese grater
- Cutting board
- Grill
- Kitchen scale
- Kitchen shears
- Knives, high-quality, sharp

- Measuring cups and spoons
- Microwave oven
- Mixing bowls
- Nonstick cookware
- Pastry brush
- Pie pan, 9 inch
- Pressure cooker
- Roasting pan with grate

- Rolling pin
- Slotted spoon
- Slow cooker
- Spatula
- Steamer
- Strainer
- Thermometer
- Wooden spoons

Cook Smart

Reliable Recipes

Recipe resources are everywhere: cookbooks, magazines, websites, and mobile apps. As you will learn in Chapter 9, some of these recipes may need to be modified to meet your diabetes needs. Still, many of today's recipes are designed for healthful eating. **When deciding which recipes to try, consider a few key points:**

- Will the recipe fit into your day's meal plan?

- Is a nutrient analysis of the recipe provided?
- Does the recipe include exotic ingredients that you might only use once or twice?
- Does the time required to cook the recipe fit into your schedule?
- Does it appeal to your sense of taste?

The American Diabetes Association's website (www.diabetes.org) is a free, rich source of recipes. It contains hundreds of recipes in categories such as "Foodie & Quick Recipes," "Budget-Friendly Recipes," "Gluten-Free Recipes," and "Vegetarian Recipes."

Batch Cooking

You may never become a master chef, but you can master the art of cooking by making the most of your time and money once you're in the kitchen. A simple way to do this is with "batch cooking"—cooking a food once and saving some (or all) of it to serve later. **Some examples of batch cooking include:**

- Make a large batch of waffles on a weekend morning then freeze them to use individually during the week.
- When preparing your evening meal, cook an extra chicken breast or two to use later in the week for chicken pot pie or quesadillas.
- Prepare a double batch of spaghetti sauce. Use some immediately then freeze the remainder to use later in stuffed peppers or lasagna.

Batch cooking is a great opportunity to stock the freezer for the days when you don't have the time to cook or don't feel like cooking. Some foods are better suited to freezing and reheating than others.

A Few Freezer-Friendly Foods

All of the following foods stand up to the freezer well. Most cooked dishes will keep for 2–3 months in the freezer.

- Baked chicken breasts
- Casseroles
- Enchiladas
- Meat loaf
- Pulled pork
- Soups and chilis
- Stuffed peppers
- Tomato sauces

A Few Freezer-Unfriendly Foods

- Fruit and vegetables with a high water content (such as watermelon or green salads) become watery and limp when frozen.
- Dishes that are yogurt-, sour cream–, milk-, or light cream–based will separate when frozen.
- Cooked pasta and macaroni may become rubbery when frozen.

Keeping It Safe

The symptoms of a food-borne illness (nausea, vomiting, diarrhea) caused by the improper storage or handling of food in the kitchen not only make you miserable, but can also have serious effects on your diabetes control. Keep your kitchen safe by properly storing, cooking, and handling your food.

The USDA recommends four easy steps to keep your foods safe:

1. **Clean.** Wash your hands, utensils, and cutting boards before and after contact with raw meat, poultry, seafood, and eggs.
2. **Separate.** Keep raw meat, poultry, and seafood away from foods that won't be cooked and use separate utensils, dishes, and cutting boards for raw food and cooked foods.
3. **Cook.** Use a food thermometer. You can't tell whether food has been safely cooked just by how it looks.
4. **Chill.** Chill leftovers and takeout foods within 2 hours, and keep the refrigerator at 40°F or below.

Got a food safety question? Visit the USDA website's (www.usda.gov) "Food Safety" page.

The Joy of Eating

"In eating we experience a certain special and indefinable well-being."
—*Jean-Anthelme Brillat-Savarin*

Food is more than just something to eat. As you deal with type 2 diabetes, you may find yourself caught up in an "eat this/don't eat that" conflict, viewing food as either "good" or "bad" rather than as a source of nourishment and enjoyment.

In the past, individuals with diabetes were told to "avoid concentrated sweets," such as sugar, candy, and desserts, because it was felt that sugar sent blood glucose levels sky high. More recent scientific evidence shows that carbohydrates (sugars and starches) have the most influence on blood glucose levels after

Looking for More Free Resources on Smart Savings and Healthy Eating?

Visit the "Healthy Eating on a Budget" page of the ChooseMyPlate website (www.choosemyplate.gov). There you'll learn how to:

- Create a Grocery Game Plan
- Shop Smart to Fill Your Cart
- Prepare Healthy Meals

You will also find sample 2-week menus designed to help you meet nutrition needs on a budget.

meals/snacks, leading to new nutrition advice: sugar can be substituted for other carbohydrates in the meal plan, as long as blood glucose is controlled and the nutrition plan is balanced.

So, take the time to savor your food and enjoy quality, not quantity. Focus on what to eat instead of what not to eat. Eat less, but eat better. Enjoy what you prepare and the experience of sharing it with others.

Next Steps

- Check your calendar to see where you'll be at dinnertime every night next week.
- Plan menus for three dinners to serve next week.
- Don't forget to savor the joy of eating!

What Do I Eat for Dinner?

FOR 45–60 GRAMS OF CARBOHYDRATE*
3 ounces marinated, grilled flank steak
1 cup fresh green beans
1 grilled tomato with oregano
Recipe: Banana "Soft Serve" (1 serving)

FOR 60–75 GRAMS OF CARBOHYDRATE*
3 ounces marinated, grilled flank steak
1 cup fresh green beans
1/2 cup roasted or grilled red-skin potato slices
1 grilled tomato with oregano
Recipe: Banana "Soft Serve" (1 serving)

*For most women, 45–60 grams of carbohydrate at a meal is a good starting point; for most men, 60–75 grams of carbohydrate per meal is appropriate. Check with your diabetes health-care team to find the amount of carbohydrate that's right for you.

Swift, Simple Tips

- Ideally, flank steak should marinate overnight for best taste and tenderness. But if you're caught in a time crunch, marinating it for 2 hours in a resealable zip-top plastic bag will work almost as well.
- Instead of salt and pepper, season the potato slices with an unexpected flavor, such as basil, cilantro, rosemary, onion powder, garlic powder, lemon pepper, or a light drizzle of fresh lemon juice and olive oil.

Banana "Soft Serve" (3 Ways)

BASIC BANANA HONEY

SERVES: 3
SERVING SIZE: 1/2 cup

PREPARATION TIME: 10 minutes
FREEZING TIME: 3–4 hours

INGREDIENTS

3 very ripe bananas (about 7 inches in length; use of ripe bananas is key for recipe to turn out)

1 1/2 teaspoons honey

1. Peel bananas and cut into 1-inch chunks. Place in a single layer in an 8 × 8-inch or 9 × 13-inch pan and freeze until frozen solid (may take 3–4 hours).

2. Place half of bananas in a blender, drizzle evenly with honey, add remaining bananas, and pulse blender. Stop blender frequently and push chunks to the bottom of the blender with a spatula as mixture will initially be very chunky and difficult to blend. Continue stopping blender, pushing mixture down with spatula, and pulse blending. With continued blending, the texture will become smooth and creamy, and the mixture will take on the consistency of soft serve ice cream.

3. Store in an airtight container in freezer. Before serving, soften at room temperature as you would ice cream, if desired.

CHOICES/EXCHANGES	BASIC NUTRITIONAL VALUES			
2 Fruit	**Calories**	110	**Potassium**	405 mg
	Calories from Fat	0	**Total Carbohydrate**	28 g
	Total Fat	0.0 g	Dietary Fiber	3 g
	Saturated Fat	0.0 g	Sugars	17 g
	Trans Fat	0.0 g	**Protein**	1 g
	Cholesterol	0 mg	**Phosphorus**	25 mg
	Sodium	0 mg		

PEANUT BUTTER BANANA

SERVES: 3

SERVING SIZE: 1/2 cup

PREPARATION TIME: 10 minutes

FREEZING TIME: 3–4 hours

INGREDIENTS

3 very ripe bananas (about 7 inches in length; use of ripe bananas is key for recipe to turn out)

2 tablespoons peanut butter (crunchy or smooth; both work equally well)

1. Peel bananas and cut into 1-inch chunks. Place in a single layer in an 8 × 8-inch or 9 × 13-inch pan and freeze until frozen solid (may take 3–4 hours).

2. Place half of bananas in a blender, dollop with peanut butter, and add remaining bananas (this layering assists in ease of blending). Pulse blend, stopping blender frequently to push chunks to the bottom of the blender with a spatula as mixture will initially be very chunky and difficult to blend. Continue stopping blender, pushing mixture down with spatula, and pulse blending. With continued blending, the texture will become smooth and creamy, and the mixture will take on the consistency of soft serve ice cream.

3. Store in an airtight container in freezer. Before serving, soften at room temperature as you would ice cream, if desired.

CHOICES/EXCHANGES
2 Fruit, 1 Fat

BASIC NUTRITIONAL VALUES

Calories	160	**Potassium**	470 mg
Calories from Fat	50	**Total Carbohydrate**	28 g
Total Fat	6.0 g	Dietary Fiber	4 g
Saturated Fat	1.2 g	Sugars	15 g
Trans Fat	0.0 g	**Protein**	4 g
Cholesterol	0 mg	**Phosphorus**	65 mg
Sodium	50 mg		

CHOCOLATE CHIP BANANA

SERVES: 3

SERVING SIZE: 1/2 cup

PREPARATION TIME: 10 minutes

FREEZING TIME: 3–4 hours

INGREDIENTS

3 very ripe bananas (about 7 inches in length; use of ripe bananas is key for recipe to turn out)

1/4 teaspoon almond extract

1 tablespoon mini milk chocolate chips

1. Peel bananas and cut into 1-inch chunks. Place in single layer in an 8 × 8-inch or 9 × 13-inch pan and freeze until frozen solid (may take 3–4 hours).

2. Place half of bananas in blender, drizzle evenly with almond extract, add remaining bananas, and pulse blender. Stop blender frequently and push chunks to the bottom of the blender with a spatula as mixture will initially be very chunky and difficult to blend. Continue stopping blender, pushing mixture down with spatula, and pulse blending. With continued blending, the texture will become smooth and creamy, and the mixture will take on the consistency of soft serve ice cream. Stir in chocolate chips (do not blend).

3. Store in an airtight container in freezer. Before serving, soften at room temperature as you would ice cream, if desired.

Recipe Tip

- If you find it difficult to get the Banana Soft Serve recipes to a smooth consistency, let the mixture soften a bit at room temperature then blend again until smooth. Works every time!

CHOICES/EXCHANGES

2 Fruit

BASIC NUTRITIONAL VALUES

Calories	130		**Potassium**	420 mg
Calories from Fat	20		**Total Carbohydrate**	29 g
Total Fat	2.0 g		Dietary Fiber	3 g
Saturated Fat	1.0 g		Sugars	16 g
Trans Fat	0.0 g		**Protein**	1 g
Cholesterol	0 mg		**Phosphorus**	30 mg
Sodium	0 mg			

Food for Thought

- Take the time to plan ahead for meals and snacks to improve your health and your budget.
- Minimize the minutes you spend in the grocery store by using a shopping list.
- Planned overs and batch cooking can help you make the most of your time in the kitchen.

I t's 8:00 A.M. You're late to a meeting and didn't have time to prepare breakfast at home, so you pull into a fast-food drive-thru to grab a quick breakfast—after all, you're hungry and know that you need some fuel. A bacon, egg, and cheese biscuit and a medium orange juice are what you order. *Seventy-one grams of carbohydrate, half a day's worth of fat, and just over 600 calories later, you're wondering if you should have made a different choice.*

No doubt, eating out is convenient and is often a social experience. Recent reports show that most Americans eat out at least once a week—more frequently at lunch than the evening meal—and in 2014, one-third of Americans' total calories came from eating outside the home. Interestingly, also in 2014, consumers noted that they planned to dine out less often because of concerns about health. Does managing diabetes mean an end to eating out? Of course not! It is certainly possible to eat away from home and still manage your blood glucose and weight. In fact, many restaurants are now trying to meet diners' needs as more diners are requesting healthy food choices, whether they are lower-fat, lower-calorie, or lower-carbohydrate options.

Planning Ahead Pays Off: 4 Strategies

With a little forethought, eating out can be as healthy as it is tasty when you implement a few smart-eating strategies.

STRATEGY #1: Try to limit dining out impulsively. Granted, "life happens," and forethought isn't always possible. But when planning ahead *is* possible, you can select restaurants with a variety of choices, thus increasing your chances of finding foods that fit both your tastes and diabetes meal plan.

STRATEGY #2: Keep two or three "go-to" restaurants top of mind. That's a favorite tip patients have shared over the years. By having two or three go-to restaurants in mind, which you know have menu options that work for you, when the question "Where should we meet to eat?" arises, you are armed with several options to suggest.

STRATEGY #3: Do some restaurant research. With even a couple of minutes notice you can gather information on your dining options and locate healthy options that best fit your calorie, fat, and carbohydrate needs. Otherwise, when your stomach is growling and your defenses are down, "everything looks good." **Here are a few quick restaurant research options:**

- **Google the restaurant and check out the menu online** to identify menu items that suit your tastes and health needs. Establishments with 20 or more locations *must* have the nutrition information available. You'll often find nutrition information posted on the restaurant's website. Restaurants with fewer than 20 locations may opt-in to share nutrition information also.
- **Use one of a multitude of free mobile apps** to check out the nutrition profile of menu offerings.

Alternatively, if time is on your side and you're giving some forethought to dining out, here are a few more considerations:

- **Invest in a guidebook to dining out** to learn more about making healthy selections at different restaurants. For example, check out the American Diabetes Association's resource *Eat Out, Eat Well: The Guide to Eating Healthy in Any Restaurant* by Hope Warshaw.
- **Request nutrition information from those restaurants you visit frequently.** Many restaurant chains have pamphlets with all the facts and figures you need, which can be especially helpful if you don't go online frequently. If you're considering a restaurant you haven't dined at before, call ahead to see what's on the menu.
- **Check out the nutrition information for many popular restaurants through a free online database,** such as www.calorieking.com.

Proposed food regulations indicate that the focus on the availability of nutrition information for menu offerings at restaurants will only continue to increase in the future.

STRATEGY #4: Always be prepared. With all of the focus on food, don't forget as you head out the door to grab your blood glucose monitor (if you have one), any diabetes medication you need to take with the meal, and any other diabetes supplies you may need. A zip-top plastic bag, small

Face the Figures

Just *one* fast-food meal can contain close to an *entire day's* worth of carbohydrate and fat. Take a look at this example:

Food items	Calories	Carbohydrate (grams)	Fat (grams)
Crispy chicken sandwich with lettuce, tomato, pickle, and mayonnaise	510	54	20
Baked potato with sour cream and chives	320	63	4
Small chocolate shake	340	56	9
Totals	1170	173	33

cosmetics bag, or small cooler bag is a simple way to transport everything together.

Dash 'N' Dine?
8 Tips to Navigating Fast-Food Dining

It's been said that the fastest-growing appliance in America is not the microwave, but the power window, thanks to the rising frequency of people eating on the run. How likely is it that you, too, will drive through a fast-food restaurant, grab a takeout meal, visit a food truck, or order food to be delivered to your home sometime in the next week? two weeks? month?

When it comes to eating on the run, here are a few helpful hints to guide your choices:

1. **Slow it down.** You may get your food fast, but slow down when it comes to eating.

Try taking two or three 1-minute "time outs" to allow your body time to realize you're getting full. Eat for 3–4 minutes, and then take a time out for 1 minute.

2. **Keep it simple.** Stick with foods in their simplest forms, such as a grilled chicken sandwich rather than processed chicken nuggets.

3. **Go easy on the condiments.** Just one packet of mayonnaise (about 2 teaspoons) adds 60 calories and 7 grams of fat! Ask if reduced-fat condiments are available. Keep in mind that "honey glazed," "honey mustard," and "barbecued" mean extra carbohydrate.

4. **Boycott the breading.** When possible, choose foods that are not breaded or peel off the breading to remove extra carbohydrate (and fat, if it's fried). We've heard patients often say they leave off the top

or bottom bun on a sandwich to trim carbohydrate and meet their goals.

5. **Eat like a child.** Kids' meals are a more favorable option for "kids of all ages" as opposed to "value" or combo meal deals. The carbohydrate content and calories in "kids' meals" are generally much closer to adult mealtime carbohydrate and calorie targets than those in "value" or combo meal deals. **If you find yourself in a fast food restaurant and need an easy answer, order the kid-size meal.** Here are some other tips to help you control fast-food portions:

    • Menu items labeled "small," "plain," and "regular" are typically the best choices for your health, whereas selections labeled "deluxe," "biggie," or "value" mean larger portions and more calories, carbohydrate, fat, and salt.

    • Select items on "right price, right size" or "dollar" menus *may* be considerations as well, given that portion sizes are generally smaller on these menus. But if you eat two of those smaller-size sandwiches, for instance, you've defeated your portion control efforts!

6. **Ask yourself, "Is a value meal really a value?"** A "value meal" is not a value when it contains more food than you need plus empty calories and excess carbohydrate. Sure, you may get more food for that extra $0.69–0.99, but, on average, you're also buying about 500 extra calories (see "Is a Value Meal Really a Value?"), which can translate over time into unwanted weight gain and associated health-care costs. A value meal generally runs about 1,000 calories or higher!

If you feel compelled to order off the value menu, try these tips:

• Share your fries with a dining companion. Alternatively, eat a few and toss the rest or take the rest home to reheat and enjoy at another meal.

• Switch out the fries for a green salad or fruit side option (now widely available at fast-food establishments). That one switch saves nearly 40–45 grams of carbohydrate and nearly 400 calories.

7. **Keep salads healthy.** Have you ever ordered a salad at a quick service restaurant thinking, "It's a salad, so it has to be healthy for me?" Salads seem like a healthy choice, and often are. There are many scrumptious salad alternatives to the traditional burger and fries. **However, loaded salads can bring some surprises. Did you know that . . .**

• A fast-food taco salad tips in at about 800–1,000 calories and 70 grams of carbohydrate?

• A chicken strip salad (depending on the size and even without dressing) runs 500–1,100 calories and 45–70 grams of carbohydrate. Just because "it's a salad" and it has chicken does not always mean it's good for you.

Is a Value Meal Really a Value?

"Value meal"		"Kids' meal"	
Quarter-pound burger with cheese Medium fries Diet soda		Cheeseburger Small fries Diet soda	
990 calories	94 g carbohydrate	510 calories	54 g carbohydrate

Takeaway: Choosing a "kids' meal" instead of a "value meal" = savings of nearly 500 calories and 40 grams of carbohydrate!

Here are some pointers to help you keep your salads healthy:

- Stick with those that are full of lettuce/salad greens and veggies, lean protein (like grilled chicken, salmon, or beans), and drizzled with low-calorie or vinaigrette dressings.
- Go easy on high-fat and crunchy toppings such as bacon, cheese, croutons, tortilla chips, fried noodles, nuts, and regular dressings. They can quickly sabotage your "healthy" salad and your diabetes nutrition goals.

8. **Pizza pointers: The thinner the crust, the lower the carbohydrate count.** If you're craving a slice of pizza once in a while, here are some pointers to help fit pizza into your meal plan:
    - Choose thin crust over original crust when ordering pizza. The thinner the crust, the lower the carbohydrate count (see Table 6.1).
    - Limit meat toppings; pile on the veggies instead to reduce fat (see Table 6.1).

Best Bets: Fast Food

Cruising through the drive-thru and wondering what to order? Here are a few of the best bets.

Fast-Food Breakfast Best Bets

- Oatmeal
- Fruit and yogurt parfait
- English muffin with margarine
- Egg white on english muffin breakfast sandwich
- Breakfast sandwich on an english muffin instead of a biscuit or croissant
- Low-fat milk, hot tea, or coffee to drink. Here are a few things to keep in mind when choosing a breakfast drink:
  - Fruit juice portions at restaurants are often excessive and typically

Table 6.1 Pizza Comparison	
Type of pizza	**Carbohydrate or fat content**
Thin crust vs. original crust	
2 slices of 12-inch **original-crust** cheese pizza	52 grams of carbohydrate
2 slices of 12-inch **thin-crust** cheese pizza	44 grams of carbohydrate
Meat vs. vegetable toppings	
2 slices of 12-inch original crust **meat** pizza	32 grams of fat
2 slices of 12-inch original crust **pepperoni** pizza	20 grams of fat
2 slices of 12-inch original crust **vegetable** pizza	14 grams of fat

30–40 grams of carbohydrate or more, which can "use up" a majority of your carbohydrate budget for the meal.

○ Black coffee or plain hot tea are calorie and carbohydrate free.

However, "doctoring them up" with whole milk/cream, sweeteners, syrups, and whipped topping not only ups the flavor factor, but also ups the calories, carbohydrate, and fat content (see Table 6.2).

Table 6.2 Coffee Comparison at a Glance			
Type of coffee drink (12 ounces; "tall")	**Calories**	**Carbohydrate (grams)**	**Fat (grams)**
Black coffee (or with low-calorie sweetener)	0	0	0
Caramel macchiato: with whole milk with fat-free milk	 200 95	 24 17.5	 8 0.5
Caffe latte: with whole milk with fat-free milk	 180 65	 14 9.5	 9 0

> ## Tips for A More Healthful Coffee Drink:
>
> 1. Opt for fat-free milk.
> 2. Switch to sugar-free syrup if your coffee drink has a flavored syrup.
> 3. Hold the whipped cream.

Fast-Food Lunch and Dinner Best Bets

Here are a few of the healthier options for each fast-food category:

- **Deli sandwich/sub:** Choose a turkey, lean ham, or lean roast beef sub on whole-wheat with raw veggies of choice and mustard (spicy or yellow). Choose a 6-inch sub over the footlong version.
- **Chicken:** Try a grilled chicken sandwich with lettuce, tomato, pickle, and light mayo. Choose a multigrain bun if possible.
- **Burger:** Have a junior or kid-size hamburger without cheese or mayo with kid-size small fries, a fruit side, or a green side salad with low-fat dressing. Choose a veggie burger if available.
- **Pizza:** Go with thin-crust veggie pizza. Opt for ham, canadian bacon, or chicken if one meat topping is desired.
- **Mexican:** Order soft shell over crispy (soft taco or burrito over chalupa, crunchy taco, or chimichanga). Opt for a veggie and bean or chicken burrito. Choose black beans over refried. Limit sour cream and cheese. Watch bean, rice, and tortilla chip portions because carbohydrate adds up quickly.
  - 1/2 cup refried or black beans = 15 grams of carbohydrate
  - 1/2 cup rice = 23 grams of carbohydrate
  - Tortilla chips = about 1 gram of carbohydrate per chip
- **Asian:** Many Asian foods are quite high in sodium, fat, carbohydrate, and calories, so portion control and selection are important.
  - **Steer clear** of fried entrées with sweet sauces (such as sweet & sour chicken or General Tso's chicken), which are high in fat and carbohydrate. Noodle-based dishes such as chow mein and lo mein are high in carbohydrate, fat, and calories too.
  - **Choose** dishes that are rich in vegetables and lean meats (such as fish, shrimp, scallops, chicken, lean beef, and tofu, as long as they are not

deep-fried). Vegetable-based entrées can be healthy choices if they are steamed or stir-fried. Shrimp with garlic sauce, moo goo gai pan, and stir-fried mixed vegetables with tofu tend to be among the healthier options.

- ○ **Go for brown rice over white or fried rice;** monitor rice portions either way. A 1/2-pint (1-cup) carry-out container of rice equals 45 grams of carbohydrate.

For more restaurant best bets, see Table 6.3.

Have a Seat: 16 In-Restaurant Dining Tips

Surely it must have been a burned-out cook who said, "I'm making my favorite thing for dinner tonight—a reservation!" Getting out of the kitchen to enjoy a restaurant meal can be the highlight of the week. Here are some strategies to keep eating out pleasurable, without sabotaging your diabetes meal plan:

1. **Think ahead.** To avoid waiting for a table, make a reservation or try to avoid

Table 6.3	Restaurant Best Bets
Appetizers	• Shrimp or crab cocktail • Bruschetta • Hummus or baba ganoush with fresh veggies • Lettuce wraps • Edamame • California roll • Seared ahi tuna
Salads	• Lettuce or other salad greens and vegetables • Low-fat dressing on the side • Olive oil and balsamic vinegar with a squeeze of fresh lemon as dressing
Sides	• Steamed, boiled, lightly sautéed, or grilled veggies • Keep portion sizes of potatoes, rice, and noodles in check
Entrées	• Grilled, broiled, baked, or roasted fish, poultry, lean meat, or seafood • Sauces on the side • Vegetarian dishes that go easy on cheese and/or sauces
Desserts	• Fresh fruit • Sorbet • Bite-size mini desserts • Cappuccino

times when the restaurant is busiest. If you take diabetes medicines, think about when you'll eat so you can time your medication accordingly.

2. **Take it easy on the bread basket (and chip basket, too!).** Just one roll, one slice of bread, or 15–20 tortilla chips can add up to 15–20 grams of carbohydrate. Decide beforehand whether it's worth "spending" that much carbohydrate before you even start your meal. (If it's a basket of steaming, fresh-baked rolls, you may decide it's worth it.)

3. **Learn to speak the language.** Knowing menu terms and cooking basics makes ordering foods easier. Scan the menu for options that are "grilled," "steamed," "broiled," or "baked." Skip "fried" or "breaded" options. Often, foods that are prepared simply (such as steamed, broiled, or grilled items) are lower in fat and calories.

4. **Do ask, do tell.** If you don't know what's in a dish or are not sure of the serving size, just ask the server to clarify.

5. **Practice meat mindfulness.** Order the smallest and leanest cut of meat on the menu, such as a 4-ounce filet rather than a 10-ounce serving of prime rib. Alternatively, split a meat main dish with a dining companion or take half home for tomorrow's lunch.

6. **Use dining out as an opportunity to get a fish serving.** Over our years in practice we've heard many patients share that they use dining out as an opportunity to work in one of those two or more weekly fish servings (that they may not desire or feel confident enough to prepare at home). Their go-to order is grilled, broiled, or blackened fish with a green salad and a nonstarchy vegetable side. There is no thinking or carb counting required, as they know this meal is

Questions to Ask When Ordering

- Is the soup broth based or cream based? (Go with broth-based soups.)
- How is the meat cooked? Is it prepared with butter, oil, or some other fat? Can the chef go light on that?
- How are the sauces prepared? Can they be served on the side?
- How are the vegetables seasoned? If they are salted, can the salt be left off?
- Can the salad dressing be served on the side?
- What desserts do you offer? Are bite-size desserts an option?

By deciding in advance whether you'd like to enjoy a dessert or not, you can order the rest of your meal and allocate carbohydrate accordingly to fit the dessert in.

well within their mealtime carbohydrate target!

7. **Order creatively.** Instead of a dinner entrée, try a salad with a small, light appetizer or a sushi roll (you can order a sushi roll with cooked fish/seafood, if preferred, as not all sushi is raw). Some appetizer/small-plate favorites to consider:

   - Shrimp or crab cocktail
   - Bruschetta (a toasted or grilled piece of bread rubbed with garlic and topped with tomatoes, olive oil, and seasonings such as basil or balsamic vinegar)
   - Hummus (a chickpea dip made with tahini, olive oil, lemon juice, salt, and garlic) with fresh veggies
   - Baba ganoush (a roasted eggplant dip) with fresh veggies
   - Lettuce wraps
   - Edamame (boiled green soybeans in the pod)
   - California roll (sushi roll containing cucumber, crab, and avocado)
   - Seared ahi tuna

8. **Substitution, please.** Ask for a substitution if a food doesn't fit into your plan. Instead of the carbohydrate-rich rice or large potato that accompanies your meal, ask for a double order of nonstarchy vegetables, which are lower in carbohydrate. Ask for low-fat

Special Order!

Feel free to make special requests so you can enjoy your meal without feeling guilty or compromising your blood glucose and nutrition goals.

Are you on a low-salt/low-sodium meal plan?

Ask that no salt be added to your food.

Are you trying to limit fats?

Ask that less or no extra butter or oil be added to your food, or that components of the usual order are omitted (such as butter and/or cheese on an egg english muffin breakfast sandwich).

Are you watching calories and fat?

Ask that sauces and dressings be served on the side. Drizzle on an amount that fits your meal plan or dip your fork in the sauce or dressing and then spear your salad or meat. Also, inquire whether your meat, poultry, or fish can be grilled instead of fried.

salad dressing rather than the regular variety or request olive oil and balsamic vinegar to drizzle over your salad. Instead of high-fat sour cream, ask for salsa on your burrito or baked potato. If you can't get a substitution, then ask that the food be left off your plate so you can avoid temptation. You're just doing what it takes to stay committed to your diabetes meal plan.

9. **Alcohol: Moderation is the mantra.** The American Diabetes Association nutrition recommendations advise that people with diabetes limit alcohol. Women who choose to drink alcohol should limit alcohol to one serving or less per day. Men who choose to drink alcohol should limit their consumption to no more than two servings per day. Alcohol has no nutritional value and may disrupt your blood glucose control, possibly causing it to drop too low. To reduce your risk of hypoglycemia (low blood glucose), particularly if you take certain diabetes medications, always drink alcohol with food. Although alcohol itself does not directly raise blood glucose, any carbohydrate in the drink (such as in mixers, beer, and wine) may raise your blood glucose. Check out Chapter 10 for more tips on safe alcohol use. Consult with your health-care team on whether and how you can safely incorporate alcohol into your diabetes-management plan.

10. **Keep it real (portion size, that is).** When your food arrives, take note of the portion sizes and corresponding carbohydrate count; then compare that count to your carbohydrate goals for the meal. Put the portion estimation tips from Chapter 3 into practice. Try to eat the same portions you eat at home

Alcohol Servings

One serving of alcohol has about 100 calories and is equal to:

- 5 ounces of dry wine or champagne
- 3 1/2 ounces of dessert wine
- 12 ounces of beer
- 1 1/2 ounces of distilled liquor (such as gin, rum, vodka, tequila, or whiskey)

Keep in mind that bartenders, and especially home bartenders, frequently serve more than these standard servings.

and use only small amounts of added fats, such as margarine, sour cream, and salad dressing.

11. **Share and share alike.** Large portions are the norm at many restaurants. Take advantage of this by sharing with a dining companion. For example, one person can order an entrée to share, such as grilled fish with vegetables, and the other can order a large green salad. Then, the two of you can share to better control portions.

12. **"To-go box, please."** Another way to turn oversized restaurant portions into right-for-you portions is to order a to-go box *when you order your meal.* Once your meal is served, immediately box up half of it so you won't be tempted to eat "just a little bit more." Now you have tomorrow's lunch or dinner already prepared.

13. **Downsize.** If you don't have a dining companion with whom you can share oversized portions or you can't tote leftovers home, then ask for a lunch-size order, half order, or child's meal to keep portions in check.

14. **Eat mindfully.** Savor every bite and pay attention to what you eat. Many people find that the first two or three bites are what bring the most taste pleasure. Try to stop eating before you actually feel full because it takes your body time to register the feeling of fullness.

15. **The Buffet One-Plate Rule.** Have you ever overeaten at a buffet (even a seemingly "healthy" one such as a salad bar)? Or gone back for a second or third plate "to get your money's worth"? Buffets can bring overeating challenges.

Try implementing the "one-plate rule," which works like this: Survey the buffet, ask yourself what items are "worth the carbohydrate and calories," grab one plate then select the items that you *really* want (factoring in the carbohydrate count) rather than piling your plate high with foods that you may not really want or need just because they're there. One plate and you're done. After all, is a second or third plate really "worth it" if it will cause you to feel stuffed and have high blood glucose after eating? Check your blood glucose 1 1/2–2 hours after eating to see the impact your portions and food choices have on your blood glucose.

16. **Dessert dilemma?** When you have diabetes, dessert isn't necessarily off limits. Sweet treats can be incorporated into the carbohydrate count of your meal plan. If you would occasionally like dessert, then compensate by reducing the other carbohydrates in your meal, such as potatoes, bread, or corn. A good approach to having your cake and eating it, too, is to order

one dessert with extra forks and share it with everyone at the table. Or order bite-size, mini desserts, which are popular on many restaurant menus. This will allow you to keep your carbohydrate in check. Or, if you've allowed enough carbohydrate to cover the dessert, enjoy the whole thing!

Remember This

Eating out is one of life's pleasures. So remember that most any food can fit into your meal plan—you just may have to adjust portion sizes. By planning ahead, making the best choices, and asking for what you need, eating out can be pleasurable and, at the same time, you can take care of your diabetes. Everyone wins!

Surviving Meal Delays

When eating out, you may end up eating later than usual or have to wait a while for a table. Here are a few tips to help you keep your blood glucose on track if your meal is delayed:

- If you know ahead of time that you will be dining later than usual, you might need a snack at the time you would normally eat the meal.
- Have treatments for hypoglycemia (low blood glucose) with you if you take diabetes medications that can cause low blood glucose. Glucose tablets are portable and easy to pull out if needed.
- If mealtime is more than 1 hour late and your blood glucose is low, treat it as reviewed in Chapter 2 or as directed by your health-care team. If your blood glucose is within your target range, but you anticipate it may go low, then eat about 15 grams of carbohydrate (such as three or four glucose tablets or a small roll from the bread basket) to prevent it from dropping too low.
- If mealtime is delayed for more than 1 1/2 hours, eat or drink a 15-gram carbohydrate snack (such as fruit, fruit juice, milk, or crackers). Consult with your health-care team on how much carbohydrate to consume for meal delays and when to take your diabetes medications.

See Chapter 7 for additional snacking guidelines and ideas. Always be prepared! Check with your health-care team to determine a game plan for these situations.

Next Steps

- Practice identifying foods at your favorite fast-food or quick-service dining venues that fit the suggested carbohydrate goals for three meals.
- Think about your favorite restaurant meals, and list two changes that you can make to these meals so they better fit your diabetes meal plan (if there's room for improvement).
- Check your blood glucose 1 1/2–2 hours after eating out and see if you're in the target range for your blood glucose levels. If not, rethink your portion sizes and carbohydrate estimations. Maybe they were off a bit?

What Do I Eat for Lunch?

FOR 45–60 GRAMS OF CARBOHYDRATE*
Recipe: Parmesan Chicken Tenders (2 pieces)
2 tablespoons honey mustard dipping sauce
Small baked potato with light margarine and chives
1 cup mixed green salad
2 teaspoons balsamic and olive oil vinaigrette

FOR 60–75 GRAMS OF CARBOHYDRATE*
Recipe: Parmesan Chicken Tenders (2 pieces)
2 tablespoons honey mustard dipping sauce
Medium baked potato with light margarine and chives
2 cups mixed green salad topped with 1/4 cup mandarin oranges and sliced almonds
1 tablespoon balsamic and olive oil vinaigrette

For most women, 45–60 grams of carbohydrate at a meal is a good starting point; for most men, 60–75 grams of carbohydrate per meal is appropriate. Check with your diabetes health-care team to find the amount of carbohydrate that's right for you.

Swift, Simple Tips

- Purchase bagged salad for a quick salad (besides lettuce, consider spinach, arugula, or chopped kale).
- Use individual, pull-top cups of mandarin oranges packed in juice. Drain, and use to top salad (if your meal plan allows).
- Microwave a baked potato while the chicken is in the final minutes of baking.

Finger Lickin' Good?

Fast-food fried chicken strips are notoriously high in fat and sodium. Check out the healthier (and yummy) make-at-home alternative, Parmesan Chicken Tenders, below. Compared to fast-food chicken strips, the Parmesan Chicken Tenders have one-third fewer calories, two-thirds less fat, and two-thirds less sodium.

Nutrient	Fast-food chicken strips (3 pieces/about 4–4.5 ounces)	Make-at-home Parmesan Chicken Tenders (2 pieces/about 4 ounces)
Calories	360	220
Total fat (g)	18	6
Sodium (mg)	990	350
Carbohydrate (g)	16	11

Fast-Food Meals for 45–60 Grams of Carbohydrate

Arby's

Classic roast beef sandwich
Apple slices side
1 potato cake and 1 packet ketchup
Water or other calorie-free beverage

Pizza Hut

2 slices of 12-inch medium Veggie Lovers
   Thin 'n Crispy pizza
Water or other calorie-free beverage

Subway

6-inch turkey sub on 9-grain wheat bread,
   with all vegetable toppings, no cheese,
   and with mustard and vinegar
1 package apple slices
Water or other calorie-free beverage

Wendy's

Large chili
Garden side salad, no croutons with vinai-
   grette dressing
Apple slices side
Water or other calorie-free beverage

PARMESAN CHICKEN TENDERS

SERVES: 8

SERVING SIZE: 2 chicken tenders
(approximately 4 ounces total)

PREPARATION TIME: 15 minutes

COOKING TIME: Approximately 25 minutes

These "faux-fried" chicken tenders are crumb coated and baked (instead of fried) until crispy.

INGREDIENTS

Nonstick cooking spray
2 egg whites
1/4 cup skim (fat-free) milk
1 cup plain fine bread crumbs
3 tablespoons reduced-fat grated
   parmesan cheese
1/4 teaspoon garlic powder
1/4 teaspoon salt
2 pounds chicken tenderloins
144 sprays of spray butter (the refrigerated
   variety, such as I Can't Believe It's Not
   Butter; use 9 sprays per chicken tender)

1. Preheat oven to 375°F.
2. Coat an 8 × 8-inch and a 9 × 13-inch baking pan with cooking spray. Set aside.
3. Place egg whites and milk in a large, shallow bowl and whisk to mix well.
4. In a zip-top plastic bag, combine bread crumbs, parmesan cheese, garlic powder, and salt. Seal bag and shake to mix well.
5. Remove any gristle from chicken tenderloins. Dip each tenderloin in the egg mixture, transfer to the zip-top bag and shake to coat well with crumbs. Repeat, coating the tenderloin a second time with the egg mixture and crumbs. Place the tenderloin in baking pan. Coat remaining tenders using the same process. (You can work in batches coating 2–3 tenderloins at a time then placing them in baking pans.)
6. Once all the tenderloins are breaded, evenly coat each with 5 sprays of spray butter. Bake uncovered on middle oven rack for 20 minutes. Take pans out of the oven. Spray each tender with 4 more

(continued on next page)

PARMESAN CHICKEN TENDERS *(Continued)*

sprays of butter. Return to the oven and bake for an additional 5 minutes, or until chicken is no longer pink when you cut into it.

7. Leftovers reheat well in the microwave (breading softens) or in an oven/toaster oven (for crisper breading).

Recipe Tips

- Find chicken tenderloins alongside other cuts of chicken in the fresh meat case or freezer section of your grocery store. You can also choose to cut fresh chicken breasts into strips.
- As an alternative to eating these as an entrée, you can dice the chicken tenders to top a green salad.
- Nestle chicken tenders in a whole-wheat flour tortilla with shredded lettuce, diced tomato, and avocado for a quick wrap.
- Serve one or two chicken tenders in a bun for a delicious chicken-strip sandwich.

CHOICES/EXCHANGES
1 Starch, 3 Lean Protein

BASIC NUTRITIONAL VALUES

Calories	220	**Potassium**	255 mg
Calories from Fat	50	**Total Carbohydrate**	11 g
Total Fat	6.0 g	Dietary Fiber	1 g
Saturated Fat	1.4 g	Sugars	1 g
Trans Fat	0.0 g	**Protein**	28 g
Cholesterol	70 mg	**Phosphorus**	230 mg
Sodium	350 mg		

Food for Thought

- **Keep two or three "go-to" restaurants top of mind.** Whether dining out is planned or unplanned, you'll have dining options in mind that have menu items that work for you.
- **Do some restaurant research.** Locate healthy options that fit your calorie, fat, and carbohydrate needs so ordering is simple.
- **Eat with your eyes wide open.** Keep an eye on portion sizes, condiments, and cooking methods in order to keep eating out pleasurable and stay in line with your diabetes meal plan.
- **"Substitution, please."** Ask for a substitution if a food doesn't fit into your meal plan or ask that the food be left off your plate to avoid temptation. You're doing what it takes to stay committed to your diabetes meal plan.

To Snack or Not to Snack?

Whether in the middle of the afternoon, before bedtime, at the desk, in front of the computer, by the television, in the car, or at a sporting event, people snack. Have you ever found yourself munching because you're bored or stressed? Have you caught yourself mindlessly snacking while watching TV? Snacks have a way of sneaking into life, whether they're planned or not.

Since discovering that you have type 2 diabetes, have you been trying to eat smaller meals with snacks in between in an attempt to regulate your blood glucose? Or have you actually cut out snacking in an attempt to lose a little weight? To snack or not to snack with type 2 diabetes? That is the question!

Snacking: Why, When, and What?

In years past, typical meal plans for type 2 diabetes often called for two or three between-meal snacks each day. It was believed that snacks were necessary to help stabilize blood glucose levels. Now we know that not everyone with diabetes (particularly type 2 diabetes) routinely needs between-meal snacks, especially if three regular meals are part of the day. Extra calories and carbohydrate from unplanned or unnecessary snacks can translate into extra pounds and higher blood glucose. However, snacks may serve several positive purposes for people with diabetes. This chapter's focus is to bring

> ## Snack Calories and Carbohydrate Count!
>
> Snacks add extra calories and carbohydrate. Count them in your meal plan accordingly. If weight loss is your goal, be sure to carefully plan the extra snack calories and extra carbohydrate into your day!

clarity to three key topics so that you can snack with success:

- **Why** to snack
- **When** to snack
- **What** to snack on

Why to Snack

Planned snacks (the key word here is "planned") may serve several purposes:

1. To curb your appetite and prevent overeating at mealtime
2. To head off hypoglycemia (low blood glucose)
3. To refuel your body between meals; when meals are delayed; and before, during, and/or after physical activity
4. To boost your calorie intake (though most adults with type 2 diabetes are trying to reduce calorie intake to manage weight)

When to Snack

As we alluded to earlier in this chapter, snack times can certainly vary from person to person. While one person may find that a late-morning nibble fuels their prelunch exercise class and helps head off hypoglycemia, another may need a small, midafternoon munchie to head off presupper starvation. And yet another may find that a few bites near bedtime work best. Listen to your body and your blood glucose levels; let them be your guide when it comes to snacking. Ask yourself these questions when considering having a snack:

- Are you truly hungry? Keep in mind that snacks add extra calories. So if weight loss is one of your goals, plan for those extra snack calories by trimming calories elsewhere in the day.
- Do you need extra fuel for physical activity?

> ## Did You Know . . .
>
> Just 1 ounce of dry-roasted peanuts (about 40 nuts) has about 160 calories? While peanuts are a low-carbohydrate snack, many people can finish off that small handful in only a few bites! Be mindful of how much you eat.

- Do you need extra carbohydrate to keep blood glucose levels on target?

If the answer is "yes" to any of these questions, then it may be time for a snack.

5 Considerations to Help Size Up When You Need a Snack

#1: Weight Goals

Do you need to lose weight, maintain weight, or gain weight?

- If you want to **lose or maintain weight,** a small, planned, between-meal snack can help curb your appetite and prevent overeating at mealtime. The key is to include the calories and carbohydrate in your daily meal plan to avoid weight gain and/or blood glucose spikes.
- If you want to **gain weight,** those extra calories from snacks can help you achieve your weight-gain goal. Keep in mind that carbohydrate still needs to be counted, though.

#2: Diabetes Medications (If Any)

If you're taking diabetes medications, are you at risk for or do you experience hypoglycemia (low blood glucose) when your medication is at peak action?

If the answer is "yes," a carbohydrate-containing snack can help you head off hypoglycemia. Keep in mind that snacks add extra

calories, so if weight loss is one of your goals, plan for those extra calories by trimming calories elsewhere in the day. **Here are some safe-snacking guidelines to consider based on whether or not you take diabetes medications:**

- **If you manage your diabetes with insulin or other diabetes medications,** mid-morning or mid-afternoon snacks may be an essential part of your meal plan to help provide energy and prevent hypoglycemia (low blood glucose). A snack at bedtime may be called for if your blood glucose levels are below target range (generally <100 mg/dL) or if your blood glucose has a tendency to drop in the middle of the night. It may also be time for a snack if you know you will be eating your next meal later than usual—that bit of extra fuel will keep your blood glucose from falling too low. Consult your diabetes health-care team to determine if you should use snacks to prevent hypoglycemia.
- **If you manage your type 2 diabetes exclusively through healthy eating and physical activity and eat regular meals,** then between-meal snacks are not routinely necessary. Your blood glucose is not likely to drop too low, because you are not taking any diabetes medications. However, a snack could be in order for appetite control if your meals are small and hunger hits mid-morning or mid-afternoon, or if you need to fuel up after extra activity.

Consult your diabetes health-care team for guidance on whether snacks are necessary for you and how to fit them into your meal plan.

#3: Blood Glucose Patterns

Does your blood glucose log show patterns of low blood glucose at certain times of day? If the answer is "yes," a snack may help head off that hypoglycemia. However, if you take diabetes medicines that can cause hypoglycemia, many health-care providers prefer to try adjusting medication doses to prevent frequent hypoglycemia rather than encouraging additional food intake, particularly if weight control is a concern. Ask your diabetes health-care team if this applies to you.

#4: Activity

Do you need extra carbohydrate to fuel physical activity and replenish your energy stores afterward?

- Extra carbohydrate is usually not needed to balance low to moderate physical activity of short duration, like a stroll around the block.
- For a higher-intensity and/or longer-duration activity, like a 30-minute jog or a one-hour Zumba or spin class, a carbohydrate snack may in fact be needed before, during, or even after physical activity.

#5: Age

Do you need extra fuel based on your age and/or appetite?

- **Children** may need to eat every 3–4 hours because they have small stomachs.
- **Teenagers** may need the extra calories from snacks during the day because they are growing and active.
- **Adults** may find that a small planned snack satisfies midday hunger, although some adults can do without snacks. During pregnancy, several small snacks may be preferable and necessary.
- **Older adults** with small appetites may find they prefer eating small meals with several snacks.

What to Snack On

When the munchies hit, you may not know what to eat. *Should you avoid fruits for snacks? Do you have to eat protein with carbohydrate for a snack? Is a cookie off limits?* The answer to all of these questions is "no!"

Before you dive into a snack, learn as much as you can about its nutrition profile and the amount of carbohydrate each serving contains (whether via the nutrition information label, a mobile app, etc., as reviewed in Chapter 2). Take a peek at the fat, sodium, and calories, and try to keep those as low as possible. Be sure to compare the standard serving size to the portion size you actually plan to eat, and count the carbohydrate accordingly.

Consider pretzels, for instance: According to the label on the food package, one serving of tiny pretzel twists is 1 ounce (20 twists), which contains 22 grams of carbohydrate. If you eat double that serving size (40 twists), then the carbohydrate doubles, too.

Unsure about whether you really need snacks or how to fit them into your meal plan for optimal blood glucose control? Talk with your diabetes health-care team about if/when to incorporate snacks to best fuel your body and keep blood glucose levels in target based on your appetite, meal plan, physical activity, diabetes medications, and blood glucose trends. To see how a food and/or beverage impacts your blood glucose, check your blood glucose 1 1/2–2 hours after eating and note the response.

Snacking Unwrapped: How Much Is Enough?

For most people with type 2 diabetes, a suitable snack typically contains 15–30 grams of carbohydrate.

Snack Myth Busters

Myth: Fruit should not be eaten as a snack.

Fact: One serving of fruit (such as a small orange) is actually a convenient, nutritious, and delicious snack! It contains about 15 grams of carbohydrate—the ideal amount for a small snack.

Myth: If you eat carbohydrate for a snack, you must eat protein with it (such as peanut butter or cheese with crackers) to keep blood glucose levels stable.

Fact: Research shows that in individuals with type 2 diabetes, protein does not increase blood glucose levels or slow the digestion of carbohydrate. Therefore, protein does not have to be eaten with a carbohydrate snack to keep blood glucose stable. Furthermore, adding protein to a carbohydrate snack *does not* aid in the prevention or treatment of hypoglycemia. A little protein may help promote the feeling of satiety, though.

Myth: Sweet treats (such as a cookie) are off limits when you have diabetes.

Fact: Current nutrition guidelines for people with diabetes conclude that sugary foods *do not* have to be avoided, but the grams of carbohydrate in sweets do have to be counted and included in your total carbohydrate count. As reviewed in Chapter 2, sugar is just one type of carbohydrate. Research shows that if the carbohydrate in a sweet treat is counted in the meal or snack and kept within goal levels (or covered with insulin or other glucose-lowering medications), then blood glucose control should not be significantly affected.

> ## Did You Know . . .
>
> One regular-size bag of microwave popcorn contains 10–12 cups of popped corn? Eat it all and you crunch down 50–60 grams of carbohydrate! (Kettle corn contains even more carbohydrate.)
>
> Snack smart by switching to "mini" or "snack-size" bags, which will cut that carbohydrate in half. You can still enjoy popcorn, but in a portion size that's better for your diabetes and waistline.

Check your blood glucose 1 1/2–2 hours after eating a snack to note the impact on your blood glucose. (If, however, the snack is used to treat hypoglycemia, recheck your blood glucose 15 minutes after eating to ensure that it has risen above 70 mg/dL. If not, re-treat with another 15 grams of carbohydrate or as instructed by your diabetes health-care team.)

Select Smart Snacks

When snack time hits, remember the 3 "S's"— Select Smart Snacks.

Select your snacks with these criteria in mind:

- Help you maintain blood glucose targets
- Promote good health
- Tasty
- Satisfying
- Easy to prepare

Selecting smart snacks begins at home. Keeping the pantry and refrigerator stocked with smart snacks means that when the munchies hit, you will be prepared. We've compiled a multitude of snack ideas gleaned from our patients with diabetes over the years. We hope you enjoy them too. **Adjust the portion sizes to fit your needs.** Snack on!

7 Smart Snacks at Home*

- Frozen grapes: Wash and dry grapes well and freeze them on a tray. Then place in a zip-top bag. They'll remind you of bites of sherbet or sorbet.
- Dill pickle spear wrapped in a slice of turkey
- Frozen 100% fruit juice bars
- Air-popped or light microwave popcorn
- Salsa with cucumber slices for dipping
- 1 piece of whole-wheat toast or 1/2 whole-wheat english muffin with trans fat–free margarine
- Avocado slices drizzled with olive oil and balsamic vinegar and a sprinkle of sunflower seeds

---

*Carbohydrate content varies. Adjust portion sizes to fit your carbohydrate goals.

7 Smart 100-Calorie Snacks*

If calories are a concern and you're trying to keep them in check, try one of these 100-calorie snacks. All of these choices range from 80–120 calories:

- 1 medium banana
- 10 large shrimp with 2 tablespoons cocktail sauce
- 2 tablespoons guacamole and 6 baked tortilla chips
- 5 olives and 1 mini Babybel light cheese
- 1/2 cup cottage cheese with 1/4 cup berries (raspberries and blueberries are favorites)
- 15 almonds
- 1/2 cup shelled edamame (green soybeans)

    Buy frozen, steam-in-the-bag, shelled edamame (widely available in the frozen vegetable section of the supermarket). Microwave according to package directions. Sprinkle lightly with garlic salt and toss to coat. Store in a zip-top bag in the refrigerator. We enjoy it as a snack, a side dish, or tossed in salads.

As an alternative to these 100-calorie snacks, you can choose one of the countless prepackaged, 100-calorie snack packs available at the supermarket. Many of these 100-calorie snack packs contain 15–20 grams of carbohydrate—just the right amount. Check out the nutrition information label to see which snack packs fit your snack nutrition needs!

7 Smart Snacks to Go*

What do you do when you're on the run and the munchies hit? Here are some ideas for portable snacks:

- Small apple or tangerine
- Hard-boiled egg
- Unsalted or lightly salted soy nuts
- Greek yogurt cup (greek yogurt is naturally lower in carbohydrate and higher in protein than traditional yogurt)
- String cheese and a few whole-grain crackers
- 1 can of low-sodium tomato or vegetable juice
- 3 graham cracker squares

7 Smart Snacks for the Workday

Do you ever get stranded at your desk with no sign of lunch in sight? Stock your desk or workspace with smart snacks that can come to your rescue. You may choose to stash small amounts and restock as needed to reduce any temptation to oversnack or snack when you're not actually hungry. Also, try to store snacks out of eyesight to further reduce that temptation.

    If you aren't able to fully supply your desk or workspace with snacks from home, don't worry! We've included a list of smart snacks you can pick up at the nearest vending machine

---

*Carbohydrate content varies. Adjust portion sizes to fit your carbohydrate goals.

(when you need a snack in a pinch) or convenience store if that's your best option.

For Your Desk or Workspace*

- Microwavable containers of vegetable or bean soup
- Applesauce cups (no sugar added)
- Fruit cups (fruit packed in juice)
- Individual packages of nuts (choose heart-healthy almonds, walnuts, pistachios, or peanuts)
- Foil packs or mini cans of water-packed tuna or salmon
- Instant oatmeal
- High-fiber cereal bars

From the Vending Machine*

- Small bag of plain pretzels
- Small bag of peanuts, almonds, or sunflower seeds
- Animal crackers
- Peanut butter or cheese sandwich crackers (whole-wheat varieties if available)
- Whole-grain cereal bars
- Wheat crackers (such as Triscuits or Wheat Thins)
- Cereal mix (such as Chex Mix)

From the Convenience Store*

- Soft pretzel (if it's huge, share half with a companion or save half for later)

- Low-fat yogurt
- Part-skim string cheese
- Protein bar
- Can of vegetable or tomato juice
- Small bag of peanuts, almonds, or sunflower seeds
- Fresh fruit

7 Smart "Free" Snacks

If you want to squash hunger without raising your blood glucose, try one of the "free" snacks that follow. They're considered "free" because they contain 5 grams or fewer of carbohydrate and fewer than 20 calories per serving.

- 1/2 cup diced tomato drizzled with 1 teaspoon fat-free italian dressing
- 1 cup sugar-free gelatin with 1 teaspoon light whipped topping
- 1/2 cup baby carrots
- 1/4 cup blackberries
- Flavor-infused water (such as the Lemony Spa Water or Watermelon Rosemary Refresher on pages 204–205)
- Mug of low-sodium broth or bouillon
- 2 homemade frozen pops made from diet soda or a sugar-free fruit drink (such as sugar-free Kool-Aid or Crystal Light)

7 Smart Two–Food Group Snacks*

Make snack time an opportunity to mix and match. Consider working with two different

---

*Carbohydrate content varies. Adjust portion sizes to fit your carbohydrate goals.

food groups to help ensure that the snack provides a variety of nutrients. (Refer back to Chapter 2 for a review of all the food groups.) Snacks are a great opportunity to work in fruit, vegetable, and milk servings. Here are some examples:

- Apple or pear slices with reduced-fat cheddar or soy cheese
- Broccoli florets and garlic hummus
- High-fiber cereal (5 or more grams of fiber per serving) with low-fat milk
- Peanut butter on a whole-grain toaster waffle
- Low-fat, no-sugar-added yogurt topped with fruit or as a dip for fruit
- Whole-grain pita chips and bean dip
- Tomato soup
- 1 date stuffed with almond butter (split date and remove the pit if necessary; stuff with almond butter)

7 Tips to Crush the Munchies

When you get the urge to munch, it's important to distinguish whether your craving is physiological or psychological. *Are you experiencing actual hunger in your stomach? Are you beginning to feel weak, shaky, or irritable from dropping blood glucose levels?* These are physical cravings that do signal the need for food. Emotions, however, play a big part in snacking, too. Feeling stressed, anxious, frustrated, or lonely can trigger the urge to snack. Even memories of how good certain foods made you feel when you were younger can send you searching for that snack.

Keep in mind, too, that sensory triggers, such as smells and visual cues, can set off cravings. If you leave foods sitting on the counter, then they can trigger the thought that something tasty would be nice. Have you found yourself wanting a snack while watching a favorite TV program? Food commercials give you subtle (or not so subtle) reminders to eat.

So, before snagging a snack, think seriously about why you want the snack and whether you really need it. To totally crunch the urge to munch (when you don't need the extra calories or carbohydrate), try the following tips:

- Pop a breath mint or breath strip
- Use a spray of breath freshener
- Chew a piece of sugar-free gum
- Rinse your mouth with mint mouthwash or brush your teeth
- Suck on ice chips
- Take a 5- or 10-minute walk
- Drink a large glass of water or another calorie-free beverage

Top 20 Snacking Strategies

1. **Plan, plan, and plan!** The best snack is one that's incorporated into your meal plan.
2. **Keep calories in check.** If you're trying to lose or maintain weight, keep an eye on the calories in the snack portions you eat.
3. **Snack with a reason.** Snack only when you're truly hungry or need extra carbohydrate to fuel physical activity or head off hypoglycemia.

4. **Don't let stress eating defeat you.**
    When the urge to nibble knocks, check
    with your stomach to see if you're truly
    hungry. Eating out of boredom or in
    response to pressure may lead to weight
    gain and rising blood glucose levels.

5. **Establish a snacking zone.** Eat only
    at the kitchen table so other locations
    won't serve as food cues. For instance,
    if you snack in the recliner in front
    of the TV, each time you sit there,
    you may find you want to munch on
    something.

6. **Do away with distractions.** It is too
    easy to mindlessly overeat while engaged
    in another activity like working on the
    computer, playing video games, watching
    a movie, or watching TV. When eating,
    eliminate distractions and focus on your
    food to help you feel satisfied more
    quickly and avoid overeating.

7. **If in doubt, keep it out.** If there's a snack
    food that's too much of a temptation
    and triggers you to overeat, keep it out
    of the house. If chips are a weakness, but
    there aren't any in the house, those fresh
    fruits or veggies in the fridge may seem
    more desirable.

8. **Out of sight, out of mind.** Keep snack
    foods out of sight so you aren't tempted
    to nibble for no reason.

9. **Make snacks count.** Make snack time an
    opportunity to work in a fruit, vegetable,
    milk/milk substitute, or whole-grain
    serving.

10. **Chill out.** When you're craving a sweet
    and cool treat, try frozen grapes or
    frozen banana chunks. They are an easy
    way to satisfy your sweet tooth and
    work in a fruit serving!

11. **Broaden your snacking horizons.** Try
    something new for snacks. Maybe it's soy
    nuts, pita bread with hummus, or jicama.

12. **Simple is as simple does.** Keep snacking
    simple and convenient. Have nutritious,
    prepared, and ready-to-eat snack options
    at your fingertips. If fruit and vegetable
    chunks are conveniently precut, pre-
    pared, and in the fridge, you might be
    more likely to grab them than if they
    have to be washed, peeled, and cut.

13. **Love those leftovers.** A small serving of
    last night's entrée or veggie could make
    an easy, tasty snack. Be sure it's a health-
    ful portion, though.

14. **Watch out for portion distortion.** What
    is commonly considered a "portion" is
    often actually more than enough. As
    reviewed earlier in this chapter, many
    people think of a bag of microwave
    popcorn as one "portion." But if you
    eat the whole bag, that one "portion"
    actually has 50–60 grams of carbo-
    hydrate. Ask yourself whether you really
    need that many calories or that much
    carbohydrate.

15. **Keep snacks snack size.** Smaller,
    carbohydrate-controlled, snack-size
    portions can curb hunger without nega-
    tively affecting blood glucose levels.

16. **Snack outside the box.** Measure snacks and put an appropriate portion in a bowl or zip-top plastic bag so you know exactly how much you are eating. If you eat directly from a large bag or box, then it's difficult to know exactly how much you've eaten. Did you just eat 52 goldfish crackers or 72? It can be hard to keep track! Studies show that when people eat from bulk-size bags, they eat more.

17. **Single size can be wise.** Buy snacks in single-serving packages to easily keep portions in check.

18. **Check out label lingo.** Don't be fooled by labeling claims. Foods marketed as "low fat" or "fat free" can still be high in calories and carbohydrate. Check the nutrition information label to find out the whole story.

19. **Make a perfect match.** Match snack calories and carbohydrate to your activity and blood glucose. A marathon runner can consume more calories and carbohydrate than someone who is sedentary.

20. **Enjoy your snack!** Choose snacks that you enjoy! If you don't like raw broccoli, then don't force yourself to eat it.

Next Steps

List three snacks you can eat at home that meet your taste and nutrition needs.

1. _____

2. _____

3. _____

List three snacks you can eat on the go that meet your taste and nutrition needs.

1. _____

2. _____

3. _____

What Do I Eat for a Snack?

**7 SMART 15-GRAM
CARBOHYDRATE SNACKS***

- 1/4 cup Rosemary Roasted Nuts (see page 129 for recipe) plus 4 dried apricot halves
- 1 cup cantaloupe
- 3/4 ounce pretzels (approximately 15 tiny twists)
- 6 ounces low-fat or fat-free yogurt
- 1 (6-inch) tortilla sprinkled lightly with reduced-fat cheddar, heated, and topped with salsa
- 1/2 large grapefruit
- 1/2 cup sugar-free pudding

**7 SMART 30-GRAM
CARBOHYDRATE SNACKS***

- 1 1/2 cups fresh pineapple
- 1/2 large (about 4-ounce) whole-wheat bagel with fat-free cream cheese
- 8 animal crackers and 1 cup low-fat milk
- 6 cups air-popped or low-fat microwave popcorn
- 1 cup mixed berries topped with 6 ounces greek yogurt
- 1/4 cup dried fruit
- 1 slice whole-wheat toast with 2 table-spoons apple butter

*For most women, 15 grams of carbohydrate at a snack is appropriate; for most men, 15–30 grams of carbohydrate is appropriate. Check with your diabetes health-care team to find the amount of carbohydrate that's right for you.

ROSEMARY ROASTED NUTS

SERVES: 20

SERVING SIZE: 1/4 cup

PREPARATION TIME: 15 minutes

COOKING TIME: 10 minutes

INGREDIENTS

1/2 cup fresh rosemary leaves (approximately 2/3 ounce on the stem; do not use dried rosemary)

1 packed tablespoon dark brown sugar

1 teaspoon kosher salt (the coarser grain is essential in this recipe; any coarse/flaky grain salt can be substituted)

1/8 teaspoon cayenne pepper, or to taste

8 ounces lightly salted peanuts

8 ounces unsalted whole almonds

8 ounces unsalted shelled pistachios

1 1/2 tablespoons light, trans fat–free buttery spread (such as Smart Balance)

Recipe Tips

- While any nuts could be used in this recipe, those included in the ingredient list are heart-healthy nuts.
- Use these nuts as a snack or toss in a green salad for added crunch and flavor.

1. Preheat oven to 375°F.

2. Finely chop rosemary leaves (do not chop stem) and place in a small bowl. Add brown sugar, kosher salt, and cayenne pepper. Using a fork, mash and stir well until ingredients are evenly mixed. Set aside.

3. Place nuts in an ungreased 9 × 13-inch baking pan. Bake 10 minutes, or until warmed through. Take care not to burn the nuts.

4. Meanwhile, melt margarine and stir well right before mixing with nuts. Drizzle margarine evenly over nuts and toss several times to coat nuts well (this step is essential to get flavoring to adhere to nuts). Sprinkle rosemary mixture over the nuts. Toss and stir until the nuts are evenly coated. (We use a metal spatula for this step.)

5. Cool nuts and store in an airtight container.

CHOICES/EXCHANGES	BASIC NUTRITIONAL VALUES			
1/2 Carbohydrate,	**Calories**	200	**Potassium**	280 mg
1 Lean Protein, 3 Fat	Calories from Fat	150	**Total Carbohydrate**	9 g
	Total Fat	17.0 g	Dietary Fiber	3 g
	Saturated Fat	2.0 g	Sugars	3 g
	Trans Fat	0.0 g	**Protein**	7 g
	Cholesterol	0 mg	**Phosphorus**	145 mg
	Sodium	135 mg		

Food for Thought

- Planned snacks can curb your appetite, head off hypoglycemia, refuel your body, and boost calorie intake.
- Not everyone with type 2 diabetes needs snacks. Do you? Consult your health-care team.
- Depending on your choices, snacks may add extra carbohydrate.
- Know why to snack, when to snack, and what to snack on . . . just for you.
- A 15–30-gram carbohydrate snack is sufficient for most people with type 2 diabetes.

While carbohydrate is the nutrient of primary focus for people with diabetes because of its direct impact on blood glucose, for general good health it's important to routinely take a step back and maintain sight of the overall eating picture.

As you learned in Chapter 1, there is no "ideal" eating pattern for people with diabetes, but rather a variety of eating patterns that can benefit blood glucose control and lower cardiovascular risk factors. Whether you choose to eat Mediterranean style, vegetarian or vegan, low fat, low carbohydrate, or follow a DASH approach, the core recommendations for overall healthy eating from the *Dietary Guidelines for Americans* provide general guidance that's good for people with diabetes, too.

As you step back and evaluate your overall eating patterns, ask yourself:

Do you avoid eating too much ...

- Saturated fat?
- Trans fat?
- Cholesterol?
- Sodium?
- Added sugars?

Do you get enough ...

- Protein?
- Dietary fiber?
- Potassium?

If you're not sure what "too much" or "enough" means, read on and you'll quickly learn!

Because maintaining heart health (including blood pressure control) and kidney health is particularly important for people with diabetes, let's delve a little deeper into the nutrients with a specific impact in those arenas, including:

- Protein
- Fats
- Dietary fiber
- Sodium
- Potassium

Protein

As you recall from Chapter 2, protein is one of the three building blocks of the foods we eat. (Carbohydrate and fat are the other two.) Protein supplies energy and helps ward off hunger. Protein also helps build, repair, and maintain body tissues. Everybody needs protein to power their bodies regardless of whether they have diabetes or not.

Which Foods Have Protein?

Protein is found in many foods. Good protein sources include meat, poultry, and fish; eggs; milk, cheese, and yogurt; soy, beans, and lentils; and nut butters. Vegetables, cereals, and grain products also contain some protein but in much smaller amounts.

An additional consideration with protein foods is that they may contain some fat. And, as you likely know, the amount of fat varies

---

Protein's 1-2-3 Punch!

Protein from the foods you eat . . .

1. **Provides energy.**
2. **Promotes the feeling of fullness and wards off hunger.**
   Find yourself getting hungry mid-morning? Try adding a little protein to your breakfast to help keep that hunger in check until lunch. Here are some **breakfast protein suggestions** to get you started:
   - Scrambled egg whites or egg substitute
   - Greek yogurt
   - Peanut butter, almond butter, or another nut butter (some of our patients eat it out of a spoon, and others spread it on whole-grain toast or english muffins)
   - Low-fat cheese melted on whole-grain toast
   - Almonds or walnuts sprinkled on cereal or yogurt
3. **Helps your body build and repair tissue** and carry out many other processes to keep you healthy.

Did You Know . . .

- The average woman's palm is about the size of a 3–4-ounce serving of meat, poultry, fish, or seafood.
- The average man's palm is about the size of a 5–6-ounce serving of meat, poultry, fish, or seafood.

depending on the food. **A good rule of thumb is to aim for 5 grams of fat or fewer per ounce of protein.** Check out the nutrition information label to learn about the fat content of proteins you eat and to look for "hidden" carbohydrate, which you'll find in many plant-based proteins sources, such as beans, veggie burgers, or hummus. Think about the protein foods you eat.

How Much Protein Is Enough?

With the popularity of 10-ounce steaks and 3-egg omelets, there is certainly no shortage of protein in the average American diet. Most Americans get plenty of protein, but could benefit from lower-fat, lower-cholesterol, and more varied protein selections to improve nutrient and health benefits. Take this into particular consideration if you choose to embrace a low-carbohydrate (and thus higher-protein) eating pattern.

The amount of protein you need depends primarily on your age, sex, and level of physical activity. While your registered dietitian/registered dietitian nutritionist and diabetes health-care team can help confirm exactly how much protein is best for you, **generally 5–6 ounces per day will cover your basic needs.** To put that in perspective, the size and thickness of an average woman's palm is about the size of a 3–4-ounce protein serving, whereas the size of the average man's palm is closer to 5–6 ounces.

Concerned about Kidney Health?

Showing signs of kidney disease? Reducing the amount of protein you eat to below the usual intake recommendation is generally not necessary because protein does not alter blood glucose control, heart disease risk, or the course of decline in kidney function. However, many considerations come into play with declines in kidney function, and your diabetes and kidney health-care teams are the experts on what's best for you.

No evidence of kidney disease? Start with the protein guidelines suggested under "How Much Protein Is Enough?" and individualize with your health-care team.

6 Protein Pointers

1. **Keep it lean.** Choose lean cuts of meat and poultry. They have less saturated fat and cholesterol than higher-fat meats, and thus are more heart healthy. (More information on fats follows later in this chapter.) Aim for 5 grams of fat or less per ounce of protein and trim away any visible fat. Keep it lean by grilling, baking, or broiling proteins and using nonstick skillets with cooking spray for "frying." **Clue words for lean cuts of meat include:**
   - "90% lean" (or higher)
   - "Chuck"
   - "Flank"
   - "Loin"
   - "Round"
   - "Tenderloin"

2. **Flip for fish at least twice a week.** Many types of fish—including halibut, herring, mackerel, salmon, sardines, trout, and tuna—are rich in heart-healthy omega-3 fats (reviewed later in this chapter). The more often you can work in fish, the better. Fried fish doesn't count, though!

3. **Go meatless a couple days a week.** Make beans, lentils, or soy products the focus of your meals. While adding variety, this will also save you money because these protein sources cost less than meat, poultry, and fish. Try black bean soup, tempeh vegetable stir-fry, or red beans and rice. Not sure about going meatless? Start with one day each week, or by beginning the week with "Meatless Mondays."

4. **Nibble on nuts, seeds, and nut butters.** A small handful of almonds, pistachios, soy nuts, or walnuts provides crunch, protein, and heart-healthy fats. Sprinkle a few pine nuts or sunflower seeds on a salad or a few crushed pecans on oatmeal or yogurt. Lightly spread a slice of whole-wheat toast with peanut butter, almond nut butter, or soy nut butter. Don't go nuts on portion sizes, though—the calories can add up quickly!

5. **Mix it up with lean, soy-based proteins.** Try soy-based meat alternatives, such as soy-based "bacon," or meatless "beef" or "sausage" crumbles. Snack on soy nuts. Toss tofu or tempeh into soups, casseroles, or stir-fries. Substitute a veggie burger at lunch. Enjoy edamame as a side or snack.

6. **Eggs to the rescue.** As a budget-friendly alternative to meat, switch in an egg. To

---

Did You Know . . .

1/4 cup of yolk-free liquid egg substitute = 1 whole egg

Cut dietary cholesterol by making this simple substitution!

Protein Myth Busters: Hypoglycemia Prevention and Treatment

Myth: You should eat protein with carbohydrate (such as peanut butter with crackers) at bedtime to prevent your blood glucose from dropping too low overnight.

Fact: Despite what you may have heard in the past, research shows that protein does *not* slow the absorption of carbohydrate to prevent hypoglycemia (low blood glucose). In fact, protein does not increase blood glucose, but does increase insulin response. So the bottom line is that adding protein to carbohydrate does not help in treating hypoglycemia or preventing subsequent hypoglycemic episodes.

---

help keep dietary cholesterol in check, eat egg yolks and whole eggs in moderation, especially since one egg yolk has as much cholesterol in it as you should eat in an entire day. Egg whites and yolk-free egg substitutes have no dietary cholesterol and little to no fat, so they are a heart-healthy alternative to whole eggs.

Fat

For the purposes of this discussion, we're talking about dietary fat (the fat that you get from foods and beverages) and the effect that dietary fat ultimately has on your blood fat levels (lipids) and overall health.

Fat is another of the three building blocks that make up the foods you eat. All fats are

---

The Roles of Fat

Fat in food . . .
- Carries flavor and nutrients
- Gives a smooth and creamy texture (such as in peanut butter)
- Makes foods tender and moist or crispy and brown

Fat in the body . . .
- Carries fat-soluble vitamins so they can be used in your body
- Supplies two fatty acids that your body needs but can't make: linoleic acid and alpha-linolenic acid
- Supplies energy in the form of calories
- Helps satisfy hunger by making you feel full

high in calories, containing more than double the calories of carbohydrate or protein on a per-gram basis. Because fats often get a bad rap (particularly in relation to weight and heart health), you may be surprised to learn that fats have important health functions. Some fat is necessary in your diet, and there are actually healthy fats.

Meet the Fats

Although fat is often referred to in a general sense, there are actually three main categories of fat:

1. **Unsaturated fats.** These are the "healthy" fats and come primarily from plant sources. (Think avocado, canola oil, corn oil, olives, and peanuts.) The two types of unsaturated fats to get familiar with are:
   - Monounsaturated fats
   - Polyunsaturated fats
2. **Saturated fats.** These are the "unhealthy" solid fats that come primarily from animal sources. (Think bacon, butter, cream cheese, and lard.)
3. **Trans fats.** These are "unhealthy" fats that are created in food processing when liquid vegetable oils are transformed into semi-solid fats. (Think stick margarine and vegetable shortening.) At the time this book was published there were efforts in place to remove the artificial trans fats created in food processing from products on the market.

See Table 8.1 for examples of each of these three types of fat.

Table 8.1	Select Examples of Each Fat Type

Monounsaturated Fats
- Avocado
- Canola oil
- Nuts (almonds, brazil, macadamia, peanuts, pecans, pistachios)
- Nut butters (almond, cashew, peanut)
- Olives
- Olive oil
- Peanut oil

Polyunsaturated Fats
- Corn oil
- English walnuts
- Flaxseed
- Pine nuts
- Pumpkin seeds
- Safflower oil
- Sesame seeds
- Soybean oil
- Sunflower seeds and oil
- Tahini (sesame paste)

Saturated Fats
- Bacon
- Butter
- Coconut milk
- Coconut oil
- Cream
- Cream cheese
- Lard
- Sour cream
- Shortening

Trans Fats
- Vegetable shortening
- Stick margarine

What Are Omega-3 Fats?

Omega-3 fat is a notable type of polyunsaturated fat with heart-health benefits. You may be familiar with omega-3 fat as the "fish fat." Fish (especially fatty fish) are indeed rich in heart-healthy omega-3 fat, so eat fish at least twice a week. (Fried fish does not count!) Omega-3 fat is not just found in fish. **Other significant food sources of omega-3 fat include:**

- Walnuts
- Flax
- Soy
- Canola oil

Eating more omega-3 fat may help reduce your risk for heart disease by decreasing total cholesterol and triglycerides.

What about Cholesterol in Foods and Beverages?

While *dietary* cholesterol (cholesterol found in foods and beverages of animal origin) is not really a fat but rather a waxy, fat-like substance, it does raise blood cholesterol levels. The main dietary culprits in raising *blood* cholesterol, however, are saturated and trans fats.

Any reduction in dietary cholesterol may be beneficial to blood cholesterol levels. Foods and beverages with an animal origin that you might focus on modifying include dairy products, cheeses, and meats.

Blood Fats (Lipids) Explained: Getting to the Heart of the Matter

If you've had your blood fat (lipid) levels checked recently, you may want to know what it all means. Table 8.2 provides a quick

10 Easy Ways to Work in More Heart-Healthy Omega-3 Fat

- Top a mini breakfast bagel with fat-free cream cheese and smoked salmon.
- Add protein to a green salad with foil-packed tuna or salmon.
- Use dining out as an opportunity to order fish if you don't want to cook fish at home. Many of our patients over the years have shared that grilled or broiled fish is their "go-to" order when dining out.
- Eat sushi with tuna or salmon once or twice a week. Don't like it raw? Request it lightly cooked or try seared ahi tuna.
- Munch on a small handful of walnuts for a snack.
- Sprinkle chopped walnuts over a high-fiber cold cereal or yogurt.
- Sprinkle ground flaxseed on oatmeal. (Check out the recipe for Quick Cranberry-Cherry Walnut Oatmeal in Chapter 2.)
- Stir ground flaxseed into moist, dark dishes such as chili, stew, or meat loaf. Our rule of thumb is 1 tablespoon of flaxseed per serving. It's likely that no one will even notice.
- Grab a handful of soy nuts for a snack.
- When oil is called for in baking, use canola oil.

5 Switches to Eat Less Cholesterol

- Use 2 egg whites in place of one whole egg (this works well in most recipes).
- Instead of half-and-half in your coffee, try fat-free half-and-half.
- Leave off cholesterol-rich organ meats including liver and foie gras.
- Instead of sautéing in butter, use an equivalent amount of olive oil.
- Instead of a ground-beef burger, try a salmon or turkey burger. (Both can be purchased premade in the frozen foods section of the supermarket for a quick option.)

Table 8.2	**Blood Fat Descriptions and Targets**	
Type of fat	**Description**	**Target**
Blood lipids	A general term to describe all fats and cholesterol in the blood.	N/A
Total cholesterol	A waxy, fat-like substance that travels in the blood; includes HDL and LDL cholesterol.	<200 mg/dL
	The body actually makes most of the cholesterol that is found in the blood, but some is absorbed from foods.	
HDL cholesterol	Cholesterol carried by high-density lipoproteins (HDL) to the liver, where it's broken down and excreted.	>40 mg/dL (men) >50 mg/dL (women)
	The "good" cholesterol.	
LDL cholesterol	Cholesterol carried by low-density lipoproteins (LDL) to the cells where it may be used.	<100 mg/dL (for people with diabetes) <70 mg/dL (for people with diabetes and cardiovascular disease)
	Too much LDL cholesterol in the blood leaves deposits on blood vessel walls, which can lead to clogged arteries and blood vessels.	
	The "bad" cholesterol.	
Triglycerides	The most common type of fat in the body. Triglycerides come from food, and the body also makes them.	<150 mg/dL

6 Lifestyle Modifications to Address High Lipids

- Eat less saturated fat, trans fat, and cholesterol.
- Eat more foods rich in omega-3 fat.
- Eat more fiber (discussed later in this chapter).
- Include foods rich in plant stanols/sterols (reviewed on the next page).
- Be more active.
- Maintain a healthy weight.

overview of the types of blood fats and the target levels for each type.

Scientific studies suggest that a diet high in saturated fats, trans fat, and cholesterol increases the risk for unhealthy levels of blood cholesterol and, therefore, heart disease. If your blood lipids are above target, the type of fat that you eat is extremely important. Further review follows later in this section on fat quality.

All Fats Are Not Created Equal

As you've seen, different fats have differing effects in your body. Just as choosing high-quality foods is key to healthy eating, so is choosing high-quality fats. High-quality fats are the "better-for-you" unsaturated fats—the plant-based fats—reviewed earlier in this section. The Mediterranean style of eating (discussed in Chapter 1) is rich in these heart-healthy, high-quality plant-based fats and may benefit blood glucose control as well, so it can be recommended as an effective alternative to a lower-fat, high-carbohydrate eating pattern.

10 Simple Switches to High-Quality Fat

- Top your morning whole-grain toast or english muffin with almond butter, cashew butter, or peanut butter rather than butter.
- Try almond milk on your morning cereal, rather than full-fat milk.
- Add avocado to a salad or drizzle avocado slices with a splash of balsamic vinegar and olive oil and a sprinkle of sunflower seeds.
- Mash and spread avocado on a sandwich instead of mayonnaise.
- Add crunch to a salad with almonds, pecans, pistachios, pumpkin seeds, toasted sesame seeds, or sunflower seeds instead of bacon.
- Rather than adding butter or bacon drippings to vegetables, try a drizzle of olive oil.
- Switch out canola oil or corn oil for lard or shortening in cooking.
- Lightly dip crusty bread in olive oil rather than slathering with butter.

Plant Stanols and Sterols: What Are They and Do You Need Them?

Plant stanols and sterols, also called "phytosterols," are natural substances found in plant foods that may help lower blood cholesterol. Sources include fruits, vegetables and vegetable oils, nuts, and seeds.

If you have high blood lipids, you may be able to modestly reduce your total and LDL cholesterol by consuming 1.6–3 grams of plant stanols or sterols per day. Because it's impossible to get enough plant stanols and sterols from natural food sources alone, food companies enrich some of their food products with these phytosterols. If the label claims that the food reduces cholesterol, read on and see if the label claims that the food is enriched with plant stanols and sterols.

Phytosterol-enriched foods include select vegetable oil spreads, mayonnaise, yogurt, milk, orange juice, cereals, and granola bars. Look for plant stanol/sterol and cholesterol-reduction label claims to help identify these products. Check the label of these phytosterol-enriched products to determine the amount of phytosterols in each serving of the food. The amount varies from one enriched food to the next. Many people choose to incorporate a variety of plant stanol– and sterol–enriched foods to achieve the goal of 1.6–3 grams daily.

- Spread on a plant-stanol-ester "buttery" spread or low-fat, trans fat–free margarine rather than butter.
- Choose olives over cheese for an evening appetizer.

Takeaway: The *quality,* or type, of fat you eat is more important than the *quantity,* or total amount, of fat you eat. To improve the quality of fat that you eat, substitute unsaturated plant-based fats for solid saturated and trans fats when possible.

How Much Fat Is Enough?

While there is definite consensus that high-quality fat is the way to go, there is no conclusive "ideal" recommended daily amount of fat. Needs vary from person to person. Think about it—fat equals calories. If you're a runner, or an otherwise highly active individual, you need more calories than someone who is sedentary. Therefore, you could potentially eat more fat (high-quality fat) than someone trying to lose weight, who may accomplish

> ## Healthy Fat Calories Add Up, Too—Moderation is the Mantra
>
> - Slather peanut butter a little lighter on your bread. Use 1 tablespoon instead of 2 tablespoons and save 100 calories!
> - Switch the buttery topping on your baked sweet potato. Use 2 tablespoons light, trans fat–free margarine spread instead of trans fat–free stick margarine and save 100 calories.

his/her health goals more effectively with a lower-fat, and thus lower-calorie, eating pattern.

A generally acceptable range for fat intake is 20–35% of total daily calories, according to the Institute of Medicine. So, doing the math, that would mean **45–78 grams of fat per day for an average 2,000 calories.** Moderation is really the mantra because all fats are high in calories. And that's an especially important consideration if you're trying to lose weight or maintain weight loss.

5 General Tips to Trim Fat and Meet Your Goals:

1. Choose lean cuts of meat and poultry and trim off visible fat. (See "Six Protein Pointers" earlier in this chapter for more protein tips.)
2. Choose low-fat and fat-free dairy products.
3. Choose baked and grilled foods more often and fried foods less often.
4. Order sauces and dressings on the side when dining out so you can control the amount that goes on your food.
5. Practice portion control. The amount of fat that you eat depends not only on what you eat, but also on how much you eat.

Get the Facts on Fat

While you're now equipped with a number of tips to improve the quality of the fats you eat, keep in mind that many foods have a combination of these different fats. The more often you emphasize the sources that are rich in unsaturated fat over saturated and trans fats, the better.

To learn about the fat content of the foods and beverages you eat and drink, turn first to nutrition information labels to familiarize yourself with the amounts and types of fats and cholesterol. If a label is not available, you can learn about the fat in a food or beverage through reliable, free online databases, Internet searches by brand, or mobile apps. Check out the serving size for the food, too. Remember, if the amount you actually eat is more like double or triple one serving, then you're eating double or triple the fat and other nutrients, too.

Summary—Fat Guidelines for People with Diabetes

- Keep total fat to 20–35% of your daily total calorie intake.
- Trim saturated fat to <10% of your total calories for heart health.
- Limit trans fat as much as possible. Avoiding it is best.
- Hold cholesterol intake to <300 mg per day.
- Eat two or more servings of fish each week (but not fried fish).
- Include 1.6–3 grams per day of plant stanols or sterols (by eating phytosterol-enriched foods) if you have high blood lipids.

Consult with a registered dietitian/registered dietitian nutritionist and your diabetes health-care team for help understanding these numbers and determining individualized goals for you.

Dietary Fiber

Dietary fiber also deserves mention because it plays an important role in promoting good health. Sometimes referred to as "roughage," dietary fiber is the indigestible portion of plant foods. Fiber is what gives plants shape. Your body cannot digest or absorb fiber, so instead of being used for energy, fiber just passes through your body. Just as fiber provides shape and bulk to plants, it bulks up the contents of your intestinal tract. While fiber is passing

5 Fiber-Rich Food Sources

- Fruits
- Vegetables
- Whole grains
- Fiber-rich cereals (those with >5 grams of fiber per serving)
- Legumes

through, it provides a number of positive health benefits:

- Fiber aids digestion.
- Fiber promotes bowel movement regularity and colon health.
- Fiber lowers the risk of some diseases, including heart disease and cancer.

It is for these health benefits that a high-fiber eating pattern is encouraged for people with diabetes (as for the general public). Mediterranean-style, vegetarian and vegan, and DASH eating patterns (all reviewed in Chapter 1) can help you achieve a fiber-rich diet.

More about Whole Grains

Whole grains are foods containing the entire grain kernel—the bran, germ, and endosperm. Familiar examples of whole grains include brown rice, oatmeal, popcorn, and quinoa. (Check out the Mediterranean Quinoa Salad recipe on page 61.)

Research has concluded that eating whole grains is not associated with improved blood glucose control in type 2 diabetes; however, it does provide other health benefits, including reducing cardiovascular disease risk. So go for more whole grains!

How Much Dietary Fiber Do You Need?

Because of the general health benefits of fiber and whole grains, people with or at high risk for type 2 diabetes should make at least half of their grains whole grains, as is recommended for the general population. Most Americans fall short on the amount of fiber and whole grains in their eating patterns. The average American gets around 15 grams of fiber per day, whereas the recommended healthy amount is 14 grams for every 1,000 calories consumed, which means **about 25 grams daily for adult women and 38 grams daily for adult men.**

The good news is that you don't have to eat huge portions of plant foods to get the daily 25–38 grams of fiber! Replacing a morning granola bar with a tasty high-fiber cereal bar (such as Fiber One bars) easily meets up to one-third of your daily fiber goal. Focus on fiber from food sources rather than supplements, and consult with your health-care team about how much fiber is right for you.

As you've seen, eating patterns rich in fiber have many health benefits. However, to recognize improvement in blood glucose, you would have to eat >50 grams of fiber per day, which isn't realistic for most people. Achieving and maintaining a fiber intake of 50 grams per day can be a challenge since fiber isn't always palatable; it's hard to consume that amount consistently on a daily basis, and eating large amounts of fiber can bring some uncomfortable side effects (including gas, bloating, and diarrhea).

Getting Your Daily Grams of Fiber

Here is an example of how you can fit your daily 25–38 grams of fiber into your meal plan:

Food	Fiber
1/2 cup raspberries at breakfast	4 grams
1 medium pear at lunch	5 grams
1 cup navy beans at dinner	19 grams
TOTAL	28 grams

Quick Tips to Increase Your Fiber Intake

1. **Make at least half of your grains whole grains.**
   - Choose 100% whole-wheat bread over white or "wheat" bread.
   - Use brown rice instead of white rice.
   - Pour breakfast cereals that are whole grain.
   - Munch on popcorn for a snack.
2. **Eat 3–5 cups of fruit and vegetables each day.**
   - If you fall short on fruits and vegetables, think 25% more. That means if you're eating 2 cups total each day, try adding 1/2 cup more (25%), working toward the goal of 3–5 cups per day.
   - Vary your fruit and vegetable choices. Choose them in different colors so you get a good mix of vitamins and minerals.
   - Drink 4 ounces (1/2 cup) of low-sodium tomato or vegetable juice for a quick and low-carbohydrate vegetable serving.
   - Add a couple of tablespoons of dried fruit to your morning oatmeal (remembering to count those extra carbs).
   - Grill vegetable kabobs as part of a barbecue meal. Favorite grilled vegetables include cherry tomatoes, mushrooms, bell peppers, zucchini, squash, and onion chunks.
3. **Eat fruits and vegetables with the peels on.**
   - A potato with the peel on has twice the fiber of a peeled potato.
   - A 4-ounce apple with skin on has double the fiber of a carbohydrate-equivalent 1/2-cup portion of unsweetened applesauce.
4. **Eat more legumes (dried beans, peas, and lentils).**
   - Add garbanzo or kidney beans to a salad.
   - Have a cup of black bean or navy bean soup at lunch.
   - Spread mashed pinto beans on a whole-wheat tortilla, sprinkle lightly with low-fat cheese, and roll up.
5. **Stick close to nature—the less processed the plant food, the more fiber it contains.**
   - A whole orange is more filling and has nearly three times more fiber than orange juice.
   - Blend fruits and vegetables in a blender rather than "juicing" them. When you "juice," you don't get the fiber that's in the whole fruits and vegetables.

> ## Tips to Tolerate Fiber
>
> - Increase your fiber intake slowly (to allow your body to adapt).
> - Drink more water and liquids (because fiber soaks up liquids).
> - Try an enzyme-based dietary supplement designed to reduce gas and bloating (such as Beano).

Soluble or Insoluble?

Although focusing on *total* daily fiber consumption is the goal for most people, the two different types of fiber deserve mention. They are soluble fiber and insoluble fiber.

Soluble fiber is a type of fiber that dissolves in water and is found in foods such as legumes, barley, oats, and nuts. Research shows that certain soluble fibers (such as those in oat bran cereal, black beans, and pinto beans) lower blood cholesterol levels and may slightly slow glucose absorption. However, most people consume so little soluble fiber that its effect on blood glucose control is fairly insignificant.

Insoluble fiber does not dissolve in water and is found in many plant foods including whole wheat, whole grains, seeds, nuts, brown rice, fruits, vegetables, and root-vegetable skins (such as potato skins). Insoluble fiber absorbs water, bulks up the stool, and sweeps matter through the colon. You may hear insoluble fiber referred to as "nature's broom." Insoluble fiber may help prevent and treat constipation, but it has no effect on blood lipids.

Your best bet is to try to get a combination of both types of fiber.

Sodium

Why the Concern about Sodium?

Too much sodium can lead to significant health problems aside from bloating and swelling. One big concern is high blood pressure, which is common among many people with type 2 diabetes. High blood pressure, in turn, may increase your risk for heart disease, stroke, and kidney disease. There is wide agreement in the health-care world that the average American's sodium intake of 3,400 mg/day (excluding sodium added from table salt) is excessive and should be reduced. For people with diabetes, as for the general public, the goal is to scale sodium down and hold your overall daily sodium intake to 2,300 mg or less. To put that in perspective, 1 teaspoon of salt contains about 2,300 mg of sodium. However, one too many shakes from the salt-shaker is not the main source of sodium in Americans' diets.

The Truth about Americans' Sodium Intake

- 77% comes from packaged and restaurant foods
- 12% is naturally occurring in foods
- 11% comes from adding salt to food while cooking or at the table

See how the sodium in processed, canned foods compares with the sodium in fresh and frozen versions.

Food	Sodium
1/2 cup canned corn, plain	175 mg
1/2 cup frozen corn, plain	1 mg
1/2 cup canned diced tomatoes	130 mg
1/2 cup fresh diced tomatoes	5 mg

You've probably picked up on the fact that the terms "sodium" and "salt" are often used interchangeably, though here's an important distinction between the two: Sodium is a natural mineral that is also a component of salt (salt = sodium + chloride). Sodium may be naturally present in foods, or sodium may make its way into foods under the guise of "salt." **Any way you look at it, less sodium and less salt is the way to go.**

Finding Sodium

Review nutrition information labels to find out the sodium content of foods; this will guide you in making lower-sodium choices.

How Much Sodium Is Too Much?

Keep your overall daily sodium intake at <2,300 mg. More than that is too much!

1 teaspoon salt = 2,300 mg of sodium

6 Pointers If Your Blood Pressure Is High:

- Further decrease your sodium to <2,300 mg/day.
- Lose weight (if overweight).
- Try a DASH-style eating pattern (reviewed in Chapter 1).
- Practice moderation when it comes to your alcohol intake (reviewed in Chapter 10).
- Move more, sit less. Aim to get at least 150 min/week of moderate-intensity aerobic physical activity (such as walking a mile in 17 minutes) spread over at least 3 days a week (as tolerated). Don't go more than 60–90 minutes straight sitting during the day—get up and move around.
- Increase potassium intake in the absence of contraindications (information on potassium is covered later in this chapter).

Talk with your diabetes health-care team about what's best for you.

Although labels may grab your attention with a claim that a food is "low sodium" or "reduced sodium," check the exact sodium content on the nutrition information panel to see how it measures up against your sodium goals. **Single servings of a food with >400 mg of sodium and entrées with >800 mg of sodium are too high in sodium.**

Sodium Claims on Labels— Breaking it Down

- **Salt/Sodium-Free:** <5 mg of sodium per serving
- **Very Low Sodium:** 35 mg of sodium or less per serving
- **Low Sodium:** 140 mg of sodium or less per serving
- **Reduced Sodium:** At least 25% less sodium than in the original product
- **Light in Sodium or Lightly Salted:** At least 50% less sodium than the regular product
- **No Salt Added or Unsalted:** No salt is added during processing, but the product is not necessarily sodium-free

Do You Savor the Flavor of Salt?

The taste for salt is an acquired taste. Just as you can become acclimated to the taste of salty foods, you can "unlearn" that taste preference just as easily—in as little as a week—as we see in many of our patients. So, over time, the less salt and sodium-rich foods you eat, the lower your salt

7 Simple Steps to Shake Down Sodium

1. **Stick close to nature.** The easiest way to contain sodium is to choose fresh, whole foods that are as close to their natural state as possible. Although small amounts of sodium are naturally present in whole foods, the content is minimal compared with that in processed foods.
2. **Choose no-salt-added** canned goods or plain frozen or steam-in-the-bag vegetables.
3. **Omit salt** from the water when cooking pasta and rice.
4. **Rinse and drain canned vegetables and beans** (if using) to remove up to 40% of the sodium.
5. **Go for fresh meat when you can.** Fresh foods are generally lower in sodium. Meats and poultry may be brined, so check the label closely. Go for fresh or frozen (not processed) poultry, pork, and lean meat rather than canned, smoked, or processed meats like luncheon meats, sausages, and corned beef.
6. **Consider your condiments.** Sodium in barbecue sauce, ketchup, salad dressing, and soy sauce adds up. Choose "lite" or reduced-sodium soy sauce and no-salt-added ketchup. Add oil and vinegar to a salad rather than bottled salad dressings, and brush meats lightly with barbecue sauce rather than pouring on the barbecue sauce.
7. **Only add salt to foods at the table.** By doing this, you'll likely use less salt and will be able to see exactly how much is added to your food (as opposed to when you season as you cook).

threshold or preference will become. You'll be able to taste the salt at lower amounts. For instance, a regular salted-top cracker may taste too salty once you acclimate to lightly salted crackers.

Resetting Your Salt Preference

While working toward "resetting" your salt preference or threshold, focus on adding in other flavorful ingredients and begin to appreciate the natural flavor of your food.

We'll never forget hearing a patient proclaim, "Wow, I never realized how flavorful green beans are. Now that I've gotten used to less salt, I am appreciating their natural flavor."

Considering a salt substitute? If you are considering using a salt substitute, such as "lite" salt, check with your doctor first. Salt substitutes generally contain potassium chloride, which can be a problem for people with certain heart conditions, kidney problems, or who take certain medications.

Sodium Lowdown

Foods that are high in sodium may not necessarily taste salty. Check out the sodium content in these foods, remembering that <2,300 mg per day is the goal:

Food	Sodium
1/4 cup salsa from a jar	389 mg
3 ounces turkey lunchmeat	660 mg
2 slices of 14-inch thin-crust cheese pizza	760 mg
1 cup canned chunky chicken noodle soup (that's not even half the can!)	850 mg
1 cup low-fat cottage cheese	918 mg
1 tablespoon soy sauce	1,005 mg

10 Flavor Boosters to Cut Back Sodium without Sacrificing Taste

1. Whisk 1/8 teaspoon of dried thyme or oregano instead of salt into scrambled eggs or egg substitutes.
2. Season mashed potatoes with 1/4–1/2 teaspoon each of dried crushed rosemary, garlic powder, and black pepper in place of salt and butter.
3. Use crushed red pepper flakes to turn up the flavor in everything from soups, to meats, to salads, or even the occasional pizza.
4. Forgo the butter, sour cream, and salt on your baked potato and drizzle instead with 1 teaspoon of olive oil mixed with a sprinkle of fresh oregano leaves.
5. Dress up your favorite oil and vinegar with 1/4–1/2 teaspoon of dried thyme.
6. Add a splash of flavor, instead of a shake of salt, with balsamic vinegar, white wine vinegar, red wine vinegar, or other flavored vinegar.
7. Finish off asparagus, broccoli, a green salad, or fish with a squeeze of fresh lemon or lime juice and fresh ground pepper.
8. Add a dash of chili powder to corn instead of salt.
9. Add aromatic ingredients, like onion, green onion, garlic, and ginger, to your dishes.
10. Sample a salt-free herb seasoning blend in place of salt.

Have you ever tried freshly ground pepper from a pepper mill in place of fine ground black pepper? The flavor difference is striking. Disposable peppermills sold prefilled with peppercorns are inexpensive and widely available in grocery stores. A flavor boost from freshly ground pepper is just a twist away.

Potassium

Research shows that eating foods high in potassium can lower blood pressure by reducing the adverse effects of sodium on blood pressure. Examples of foods rich in potassium include:

- Apricots
- Bananas
- Beans
- Greens
- Lentils
- Nuts
- Milk
- Orange juice
- Potatoes
- Prune juice
- Soybeans
- Spinach
- Sweet potatoes
- Tomatoes, tomato products, and tomato juice
- White beans
- Yogurt

Unless your doctor has advised you to limit potassium because of another health condition, include potassium-rich foods more often.

Next Steps

- Keep a record for 3–4 days of everything that you eat and drink. Take inventory of whether you could switch out some foods to improve your fat quality, trim sodium, and boost your fiber.
- Check the portion sizes of your meat servings. Are they the size of your palm?

What Do I Eat for Dinner?

FOR 45–60 GRAMS OF CARBOHYDRATE*
Recipe: Hoppin' John (1 serving)
3 ounces diced cooked chicken breast added to recipe
2 cups green salad
1 tablespoon oil and vinegar dressing

FOR 60–75 GRAMS OF CARBOHYDRATE*
Recipe: Hoppin' John (1 serving)
3 ounces diced cooked chicken breast added to recipe
2 cups green salad
1 tablespoon oil and vinegar dressing
1 1/2 cups mixed berries
1 tablespoon light whipped topping or vanilla greek yogurt

*For most women, 45–60 grams of carbohydrate at a meal is a good starting point; for most men, 60–75 grams of carbohydrate per meal is appropriate. Check with your diabetes health-care team to find the amount of carbohydrate that's right for you.

Swift, Simple Tips

- Use bagged salad greens.
- Try frozen (thawed) mixed berries with no sugar added if fresh berries are not in season.

HOPPIN' JOHN

SERVES: 5

SERVING SIZE: 1 3/4 cups (or 10 ounces)

PREPARATION TIME: 15 minutes

COOKING TIME: 15 minutes

INGREDIENTS

2 (15-ounce) cans no-salt-added black-eyed peas (or rinse and drain peas, if a no-salt-added version is unavailable)

1 (14.5-ounce) can diced tomatoes seasoned with basil, garlic, and oregano, drained

1 bag boil-in-bag brown rice

3/4 cup finely shredded part-skim mozzarella (finely shredded provides more ample coverage than a regular shred)

1 1/4 cups coarsely chopped red onion

1 1/4 cups coarsely chopped green bell pepper

1/4 cup fat-free sour cream

1. Combine black-eyed peas and drained tomatoes in a pan, stirring gently to combine. Warm over low heat, gently stirring periodically.

2. Meanwhile, cook rice according to package directions, omitting any salt. Drain well.

3. In an 8 × 12-inch serving dish, or platter of equal size, layer the rice and evenly top with pea and tomato mixture. Sprinkle evenly with cheese, onion, and bell pepper. Top with small dollops of sour cream.

Recipe Tips

- Plain, unseasoned diced tomatoes can be used instead of the basil-, garlic-, and oregano-seasoned tomatoes.
- Use a combination of red, orange, and green bell peppers for a colorful plate.
- Diced cooked chicken or low-fat smoked sausage makes a nice addition to this recipe. Just warm the protein up in the pan with the beans.
- Add a splash of heat with hot sauce.

CHOICES/EXCHANGES

2 1/2 Starch, 2 Vegetable, 1 Lean Protein

BASIC NUTRITIONAL VALUES

Calories	290	**Potassium**	590 mg
Calories from Fat	40	**Total Carbohydrate**	48 g
Total Fat	4.5 g	Dietary Fiber	8 g
Saturated Fat	2.1 g	Sugars	7 g
Trans Fat	0.0 g	**Protein**	16 g
Cholesterol	10 mg	**Phosphorus**	290 mg
Sodium	360 mg		

Food for Thought

- **Monitor protein portions** and keep them close to the size of your palm.
- **Choose lean proteins** and keep them that way by using low-fat cooking methods.
- **Choose heart-healthy monounsaturated and polyunsaturated fats** more often and minimize food sources of saturated fat, trans fat, and cholesterol.
- **Eat fish more often** (at least twice a week).
- **Aim to eat 25–38 grams of fiber each day.**
- **Keep your daily sodium intake at 2,300 mg or less.**
- **Moderation is the bottom line!**

Congratulations on your progress and your focus on diabetes nutrition! Besides setting goals, learning about the effects of carbohydrate, reading labels, and studying portion sizes, you've been given crucial information about what foods are best for you. It may have been a surprise for you to discover that the guidelines for healthy eating for people with type 2 diabetes are the same as those for everyone. A healthy meal plan:

- Includes foods such as vegetables, fruits, whole grains, legumes (beans, lentils, and peas), low-fat or fat-free milk/milk products, seafood, lean meats, and poultry, and nuts and seeds
- Limits foods that are high in sodium, solid fats, and added sugars
- Does not include trans fats
- Helps you control your blood glucose levels and meet your weight goals

You now know that your meal plan doesn't have to be "special" or make you different from your family, friends, and coworkers. Instead, the best food choices for you are also the basis of healthy eating for everyone around you. You don't need to worry about having exotic "diabetic" foods and recipes (although a good diabetes cookbook can be very valuable). And don't think that you'll have to avoid the traditional family dishes simply because you have diabetes. Although many old and loved recipes tend to be high in fat, sugar, and salt, with a few strategic changes they'll be back on your table in no time.

Earlier chapters of *What Do I Eat Now?* contain very specific information about recommendations for the ideal balance of nutrients in your meal

Recipe Changes

When changing a recipe, focus on:

- Reducing fat, sugar, and salt
- Increasing fiber and flavor

As a bonus, reducing the fat in a recipe reduces the number of calories, reducing the sugar in a recipe reduces the carbohydrate and calories, and reducing the salt can be an important strategy for improving your heart health. Increasing fiber means you'll feel fuller and experience improved digestion. And, finally, more flavor means you'll increase your enjoyment of eating!

plan. In this chapter, we'll focus on a few general guidelines for giving your recipes a healthy boost.

Getting Started with Simple Switches

It's been said that if you do what you've always done, you'll get what you've always gotten. So, if you keep eating foods that aren't the best for your health, you can't expect good diabetes control. Turn the tables on your favorite recipes and make them healthy—it really doesn't take too much effort. Here are a few simple switches to get you started:

- **Change the way you prepare a dish.** Braising, broiling, grilling, and steaming are great ways to add flavor without additional calories or fat. If you're accustomed to basting your meat or vegetables with oil or drippings, try wine, fruit juice, vegetable juice, or fat-free broth instead. Use nonstick pans or coat pans with nonstick cooking spray instead of oil to reduce fat and calories.

- **Opt out of "optional" items in your recipes.** Cut out the salt in your cooking water or high-fat sauces on vegetable dishes. Leave off nuts, coconut garnishes, and other items you might add just for appearances, such as whipped cream topping, a sprinkle of cheese, or a dollop of sour cream.

- **Cut the condiments.** Condiments such as pickles, olives, butter, mayonnaise, syrup, jelly, and mustard can have large amounts of salt, sugar, fat, and calories depending on the condiment. If you're looking to reduce sodium in a recipe, for example, use low-sodium soy sauce and use a smaller amount than the recipe calls for.

- **Eat smaller portions of foods that are high in fat, sugar, or salt.** For example, have your salad dressing on the side and dip your greens into it, rather than dumping it all over the salad. Use only one spoonful of sour cream on your baked potato rather than two. Share your dessert with everyone at the table. "Just a taste" may be all you need to satisfy your sweet tooth.

- **Consider making only one or two changes at a time to note the impact on a recipe.**

Ready, Set, Change!

This chapter is designed to help you improve the nutritional value of some of your favorite recipes. When you're trying a recipe redo, the first step is to look at each ingredient in

French Toast Turnaround

Take a look at a simple recipe for making french toast; think about some easy changes you can make to reduce the fat, sugar, and salt while increasing the fiber and flavor. Below you'll find a list of common ingredients in a french toast recipe and the possible changes you can make to the recipe. There's also a column that shows how each substitution will enable the recipe to better fit into your meal plan.

Use this:	Instead of this:	And you get:
Low-fat milk	Whole milk	Reduced fat and calories
1/4 cup egg substitute or two egg whites for each whole egg in the recipe	Whole egg	Reduced fat and calories
1/2 teaspoon salt	1 teaspoon salt	Reduced salt/sodium
Almond extract, ground cinnamon	Sugar	Reduced sugar and calories; increased flavor
100% whole-wheat bread	White bread	Increased fiber
Fresh berries, puréed fruit, or sugar-free syrup	Regular syrup	Reduced sugar and calories

Remember—make just one or two changes at a time and note the impact on the recipe.

Macaroni and Cheese Makeover

Macaroni and cheese is a classic comfort food that packs a fat and calorie punch. To start your thinking, here are several strategies that can improve the health of the recipe without losing that wonderful cheesy flavor.

Use this:	Instead of this:	And you get:
Extra-sharp, reduced-fat cheddar cheese	Full-fat (regular) cheese	Reduced fat and calories
Reduced-calorie, trans fat–free margarine	Butter	Reduced fat and calories
Skim/fat-free milk	Whole milk	Reduced fat and calories
High-fiber cereal crumbs	Dry white bread crumbs	Increased fiber
Whole-wheat or high-fiber pasta	Refined white pasta	Increased fiber
Pepper, paprika, oregano	Salt	Reduced salt/sodium and increased flavor

Remember—make just one or two changes at a time and note the impact on the recipe.

the recipe and think about its function. Is it a garnish only? Is it there to add texture? Will the food fall apart if it's not included? **It's important to make only one or two changes at a time in your recipe so you can judge the success of the change(s) in terms of both taste and health.** Remember, a small change can have a big impact. Try a few different approaches to improving your recipes, and make notes of both your successes and those not-so-great results on your recipe so you have somewhere to start when you try again.

Fixing the Fat

Many recipes won't do well in a totally fat-free world because fat carries out several important functions in our food. **Here's a review of the role of fat in foods (as discussed in Chapter 8):**

- Fat tenderizes.
- Fat adds moisture and shape to baked goods.
- Fat carries and blends flavors.
- Fat adds creaminess to sauces and dips.

- Fat gives a feeling of satiety, making you feel full after you eat.
- Fat carries fat-soluble vitamins and other nutrients.

Cook's Notes: 7 Strategies to Cut Fat

1. Use low-fat or fat-free ingredients whenever possible. For example, use fat-free sour cream, low-fat greek yogurt, or plain yogurt in dips, or low-fat milk instead of whole milk in instant pudding. Be aware that because of its high water content, fat-free margarine may not work well if you're using it to sauté vegetables or make baked goods.

2. After you make a soup or stew, refrigerate it and skim the fat off the top before reheating. Each tablespoon of fat you skim will save more than 100 calories.

3. In homemade baked goods, substitute applesauce, puréed prunes, or another puréed fruit for part of the oil. In a banana bread recipe, for example, you can replace up to half the fat with applesauce without a noticeable change in taste or texture. Commercially prepared fruit-based fat replacers can also be found with the baking ingredients in your grocery store. Remember to consider the carbohydrate content of a fat replacer.

Fried Chicken—Only Better

Fried chicken can benefit from a healthy makeover to reduce fat, calories, and sodium, while adding in some fiber.

Use this:	Instead of this:	And you get:
Skinless chicken	Chicken pieces with skin	Reduced fat and calories
1/4 cup egg substitute or two egg whites for each whole egg in the recipe	Whole egg	Reduced fat and calories
High-fiber cereal crumbs	Bread crumbs or white flour	Increased fiber
Cayenne pepper, paprika, sage	Salt	Reduced salt/sodium and increased flavor
Baking	Frying	Reduced fat and calories

Remember—make just one or two changes at a time and note the impact on the recipe.

4. Use a graham cracker crust instead of preparing a dough pie crust, which is traditionally made with lard or shortening and gets more than half of its calories from fat.

5. Reduce high-fat, high-calorie extras or toppings in your recipe, such as nuts or coconut, by half.

6. Try commercial egg substitutes, which contain less fat and cholesterol than whole eggs. Or you can use two egg whites to replace one whole egg.

7. Sauté your vegetables or meats in a nonstick skillet with wine, chicken broth, or vegetable oil cooking spray instead of butter or oil.

See Chapter 8 for more information on fat and a number of tips to help you trim fat intake and improve the quality of the fat you eat.

Fat Replacers: At a Glance

If you're watching your weight, you may be interested in using products made with fat replacers to limit your fat and calorie intake. The fat replacers currently on the market are considered safe by the U.S. Food and Drug Administration, but since most of them are relatively recent additions to our store shelves, their long-term benefits and risks still aren't known.

There are three types of fat replacers used in food products:

- **Carbohydrate-based fat replacers,** which are made from starchy food products such as corn, cereals, and grains

- **Protein-based fat replacers,** made by modifying proteins such as egg whites or whey from milk

- **Fat-based fat replacers,** which act as barriers to block fat absorption

If you are considering using a reduced-fat product, take a close look at its nutrition information label. Products made using fat replacers may have less fat and fewer calories, but some people tend to eat more of a fat-free food, thereby losing any potential calorie savings. And products using **carbohydrate-based fat replacers can increase the carbohydrate count of the food and can potentially influence your blood glucose. For example:**

- 2 tablespoons *regular* ranch salad dressing = 2 grams of carbohydrate
- 2 tablespoons *fat-free* ranch salad dressing = 7 grams of carbohydrate

Your registered dietitian/registered dietitian nutritionist (RD/RDN) or diabetes health-care team can help you decide if including products with fat replacers in your meal plan is the right choice for you. Be mindful of portion sizes and the calorie and carbohydrate content of these products.

Slashing the Sugar

Although you may be limiting sugar to control your carbohydrate intake, granulated sugar plays a significant role in recipes, and it can't always be replaced with another sweetener. Here's what granulated sugar does for your cooking:

- Sugar adds texture, color, and bulk to baked goods. Substituting other ingredients for sugar in baked goods can cause your cakes, cookies, pies, and candy to come out very differently from what you'd expect.

- Sugar helps yeast bread rise by providing food for the yeast. As the yeast grows and multiplies, it uses the sugar and releases carbon dioxide

and alcohol, which gives bread its characteristic flavor.

- Sugar provides the light brown color and crisp feel to the tops of baked goods, such as muffins and cakes.

Cook's Notes: 3 Strategies to Cut Sugar

1. In most cases, you can cut back on the added sugar in your recipe by one-fourth to one-third without a difference in the finished product. If a recipe calls for 1 cup

---

Chocolate Chip Cookie Change-Up

Chocolate chip cookies can benefit from a healthy makeover to reduce the fat and sugar content while punching up the fiber factor.

Use this:	Instead of this:	And you get:
1/2–3/4 cup chocolate chips	1 cup chocolate chips	Reduced fat, sugar, and calories
Mini chocolate chips	Full-size chocolate chips	Reduced fat, sugar, and calories
Oatmeal	A portion of plain white flour	Increased fiber
1/4 cup egg substitute or two egg whites for each whole egg in the recipe	Whole egg	Reduced fat and calories
3/4 cup sugar	1 cup sugar	Reduced sugar and calories

Remember—make just one or two changes at a time and note the impact on the recipe.

of sugar, try it with 3/4 cup and note the result.

2. Try extracts, such as almond, vanilla, or peppermint, to enhance the sweetness of a food. Allspice, cinnamon, ginger, and nutmeg also impart a sweet taste.

3. Don't totally eliminate sugar or replace it with another sweetener in a recipe where sugar is used for texture, such as in baked goods. Unless you choose a substitute sweetener that can withstand the heat of the oven, your baked goods will not turn out as expected.

Substitutes for Sugar: At a Glance

Health-conscious consumers and millions of people with diabetes are turning to low-calorie sweeteners (also know as sugar substitutes, high-intensity sweeteners, or non-nutritive sweeteners) to help them cut back on the amount of carbohydrate and number of calories they consume. Because of this, grocery stores contain thousands of products labeled "sugar free" or "diet" that claim to offer a sweet taste with fewer calories. The low-calorie sweeteners currently on the market are considered safe by the U.S. Food and Drug Administration. And the nutrition recommendations from the American Diabetes Association state that zero-calorie sweeteners have the potential to reduce your overall calorie and carbohydrate intake—when substituted for sweeteners with calories—as long as additional calories from other food sources aren't eaten to compensate.

Navigating the maze of low-calorie sweeteners can be difficult (see Chapter 2 for additional information on low-calorie sweeteners). Tables 9.1 and 9.2 provide brief summaries of the most common non-nutritive (zero-calorie) sweeteners and nutritive sweeteners (sweeteners with calories), respectively, on the market today. Including substitutes for sugar in your meal plan is an individual decision based on your personal preferences and blood glucose goals. As always, your RD/RDN or diabetes health-care team can help you decide if including sugar substitutes in your meal plan is the right choice for you.

Takeaway: Limit all added sugars. All added sugars in excessive amounts can be harmful.

Table 9.1	Non-Nutritive Sweeteners (Zero Calories)
Product	**Comments**
Acesulfame Potassium (Ace K) • Sweet One	• 200 times sweeter than sucrose (table sugar) • All the sugar can be replaced with Ace K in recipes for sauces and beverages • Doesn't lose sweetness at high heat but recipe adjustments may be needed for baked goods • More information available at www.sweetone.com

(continued on next page)

Table 9.1	Non-Nutritive Sweeteners (Zero Calories) *(Continued)*
Product	**Comments**
Advantame • Not yet marketed directly to consumers	• 20,000 times sweeter than sucrose (table sugar), 100 times sweeter than aspartame • Derived from aspartame and vanillin • More information available at www.advantame.com
Aspartame • Equal • NutraSweet	• 200 times sweeter than sucrose (table sugar) • Made from amino acids, the building blocks of protein • Loses sweetness when heated; won't provide bulk or tenderness in baked goods so recipe adjustments may be needed • More information available at www.equal.com or www.nutrasweet.com
Monk fruit extract (Luo Han Guo) • Purefruit	• 200 times sweeter than sucrose (table sugar) • More information available at www.purefruit.com
Neotame (not yet marketed directly to consumers) • Newtame	• 7,000–13,000 times sweeter than sucrose (table sugar), 30–40 times sweeter than aspartame • Made from amino acids, the building blocks of protein • Chemically similar to aspartame • More information available at www.neotame.com
Saccharin • Sugar Twin • Sweet'N Low	• 200–700 times sweeter than sucrose (table sugar) • Recipe adjustments necessary in baked goods • Sugar Twin comes in packets; Sweet'N Low comes in the form of packets, liquid, tablets, and baking mix • More information available at www.sugartwin.com or www.sweetnlow.com
Stevia • Pure Via • Truvia	• 250–300 times sweeter than sucrose (table sugar) • Derived from the South American stevia plant • Pure Via comes in granulated and liquid form; Truvia comes in granulated and baking blend form • Recipe adjustments necessary in baked goods • More information available at www.purevia.com or www.truvia.com

(continued on next page)

Table 9.1	Non-Nutritive Sweeteners (Zero Calories) *(Continued)*
Product	Comments
Sucralose • Splenda	• 600 times sweeter than sucrose (table sugar) • Made using a process that starts with sugar and converts it to a sweetener that isn't recognized by the body as carbohydrate • Can be used for cooking and baking • Comes in granulated, fiber-fortified, and brown sugar form • More information available at www.splenda.com

Table 9.2	Nutritive Sweeteners (Calories Vary)
Product	Comments
Agave	• 4 calories/gram • Commercially produced from the agave plant • Marketed as a "healthful" sweetener, but that claim has been criticized due to its very high fructose content • Use only as a substitute for, not an addition to, other refined sugars in the diet
Date sugar	• 3 calories/gram • Made from dried dates; adds a rich sweetness to recipes • Will not dissolve when added to drinks or melt like granulated sugar (which can limit its use) • Use only as a substitute for, not an addition to, other refined sugars in the diet
Fructose	• Twice as sweet as sucrose (table sugar), so less can be used to sweeten foods • 4 calories/gram • Found in fruit, fruit juice, and honey • Does not cause a rapid rise and fall in blood glucose levels • Can be used in both home food preparation and commercial products

(continued on next page)

Table 9.2	Nutritive Sweeteners (Calories Vary) *(Continued)*
Product	**Comments**
	• According to American Diabetes Association nutrition recommendations, when fructose is eaten from foods in which it naturally occurs (such as fruit), it may result in better glycemic control compared with eating sucrose or starch • It is not likely to have detrimental effects on triglycerides as long as intake is not excessive
High fructose corn syrup	• 90 times sweeter than sucrose (table sugar) • 2 calories/gram • Contains a substantial amount of glucose in addition to fructose • According to American Diabetes Association nutrition recommendations, people with diabetes should limit or avoid intake of sugar-sweetened beverages from any caloric sweetener including high fructose corn syrup to reduce risk for weight gain and worsening of their cardiometabolic risk profile
Honey	• 4 calories/gram • Made of fructose and glucose • Oldest sweetener known to man • Use only as a substitute for, not an addition to, other refined sugars in the diet
Maple syrup	• 4 calories/gram • Made of sucrose and water with some vitamins and minerals • Use only as a substitute for, not an addition to, other refined sugars in the diet
Molasses	• 3 calories/gram • Byproduct of sugar manufacturing; strong taste • Unsulphured molasses is higher in minerals and B vitamins • Use only as a substitute for, not an addition to, other refined sugars in the diet

(continued on next page)

Table 9.2	Nutritive Sweeteners (Calories Vary) *(Continued)*
Product	**Comments**
Polyols, Sugar Alcohols • Erythritol • Glycerol • Hydrogenated starch hydrolysates • Isomalt • Lactitol • Maltitol • Mannitol • Sorbitol • Xylitol	• Contain 1.5–3 calories/gram, fewer calories per gram than sugar • Not generally used in home food preparation, but can be found in commercial products such as candy, chewing gum, ice cream, baked goods, fruit spreads, breath mints, mouthwash, toothpaste, and cough drops/syrups • May be found in products labeled as "sugar free," but these products aren't necessarily carbohydrate and calorie free
Tagatose	• 1.5 calories/gram • Low in carbohydrate and similar to fructose in structure • Minimal effect on blood glucose and insulin levels • Use only as a substitute for, not an addition to, other refined sugars in the diet
Trehalose	• 4 calories/gram • Less than half as sweet as sucrose (table sugar), so used more as a preservative than a sweetener • Results in a low insulin response • Use only as a substitute for, not an addition to, other refined sugars in the diet
Turbinado sugar	• 4 calories/gram • Commonly called "sugar in the raw" • Made from pure cane-sugar extract; it looks like brown sugar but is paler in color with a subtle molasses flavor • Use only as a substitute for, not an addition to, other refined sugars in the diet

This is only a partial list of the sweeteners on the market. Check your grocery store for store brands that contain the above-mentioned ingredients but may be marketed under different names. The Calorie Control Council website (www.caloriecontrol.org) is a helpful resource for more information on sweeteners, fiber, and fat replacers.

Shake the Salt

Table salt is the oldest known food additive. Although it occurs naturally in some foods, for most people, salt sneaks into the diet from processing and preparation or from the salt-shaker at the table. Salt in foods has one of three functions:

- Salt helps preserve food.
- Salt adds flavor.
- Salt aids in the rising of yeast breads.

Because people with diabetes are at higher risk for heart disease, limiting salt intake can be an important strategy for controlling blood pressure. Uncontrolled blood pressure can also damage the kidneys.

Cook's Notes: 5 Strategies to Skip Salt

1. Try herbs and spices—such as basil, bay leaves, dill, parsley, sage, tarragon, and thyme—as replacements for salt in recipes. They work particularly well.
2. Be sure to taste your food before adding salt; removing the saltshaker from the table is a simple way to slash your salt intake.
3. Trim salt in recipes. In many recipes, the amount of salt can be cut in half or completely eliminated without much change in taste or texture.
4. Substitute lower-sodium versions of canned vegetables, soy sauce, broth, and seasoning mixes.

Clam Chowder—Only Better

A healthy makeover of clam chowder results in a better-for-you version that's lower in fat, calories, salt, and carbohydrate.

Use this:	Instead of this:	And you get:
Canadian bacon	Pork bacon	Reduced fat, calories, and salt/sodium
Skim/fat-free milk or fat-free half-and-half	Cream	Reduced fat and calories
Flour or cornstarch	A portion of the potatoes	Reduced carbohydrate and calories
Bay leaves, chives, garlic, parsley, paprika, thyme	Salt	Reduced salt/sodium and increased flavor

Remember—make just one or two changes at a time and note the impact on the recipe.

5. Cut back on high-sodium foods in your recipes. Limit bacon, ham, pickles, olives, and sauerkraut. Keep an eye on condiments, such as mustard, ketchup, and barbecue sauce, which are also significant salt sources.

Check out Chapter 8 for more information on sodium in your meal plan.

Salt Substitutes: At a Glance

People with diabetes are at a higher risk of hypertension (high blood pressure) and kidney disease. Too much salt in your meal plan can contribute to both of these issues and you may find your health-care team telling you to cut back on your salt intake. *Should you consider using a salt substitute in this situation?*

As reviewed in Chapter 8, many salt substitutes are made using potassium chloride in place of sodium chloride. Excess potassium can be harmful if you have kidney problems, certain heart conditions, or if you are taking certain medications. Salt substitutes are not a healthy option for everyone. Your RD/RDN or diabetes health-care team can help you decide if including a salt substitute in your meal plan is the right choice for you.

For some people, the bitter taste of salt substitutes can also be a concern. There are other alternatives to salt that are simply salt-free seasoning blends made from different herbs and spices. You can enjoy those without concern.

Keep in mind, as discussed in Chapter 8, that the taste for salt is an acquired one, so it can also be unlearned. Most of the sodium we eat isn't from the saltshaker, but comes from processed foods and restaurant meals. As always, carefully read the nutrition information labels on the foods you eat to help you make lower-sodium choices.

Fiber Up!

Fiber is loaded with health benefits (as discussed in Chapter 8)! **In our bodies, fiber works to:**

- improve digestion and colon health
- lower the risk of heart disease and cancer

Because most Americans get less than half the daily recommended amount of fiber, packing your recipes with a fiber punch is a good strategy for better health.

Cook's Notes: 4 Strategies to Fill In with Fiber

1. Use whole-wheat flour to replace one-quarter to one-half of the all-purpose flour in most recipes.
2. Choose whole-grain or high-fiber pasta, brown rice, and whole-grain cereals as recipe ingredients. The goal is to make half your grains whole grains.
3. Add extra vegetables to your recipes whenever you can. Pasta, casseroles, and soups can be enhanced easily with colorful, high-fiber vegetables.
4. Bring on the beans! Both dried beans and canned beans are an excellent source of fiber (**just drain and rinse canned beans to remove up to 40% of the extra sodium from processing**).

Maximized Muffins

Switching out a few ingredients through a muffin "makeover" may yield muffins that are reduced in sugar, calories, salt, and fat, yet maximized in fiber and flavor.

Use this:	Instead of this:	And you get:
1 cup all-purpose flour plus 1 cup 100% whole-wheat flour	2 cups all-purpose flour	Increased fiber
3/4 cup sugar	1 1/2 cups sugar	Reduced sugar and calories
1/4 teaspoon salt	1/2 teaspoon salt	Reduced salt/sodium
3/4 cup egg substitute or 6 egg whites (2 for each whole egg in the recipe)	3 whole eggs	Reduced fat and calories
1/2 cup canola or corn oil plus 1/2 cup unsweetened applesauce	1 cup oil	Reduced fat and calories
1/4 cup coconut	1/2 cup coconut	Reduced fat and calories
2 teaspoons vanilla extract	1 teaspoon vanilla extract	Increased flavor
2 cups chopped apples with peels on	2 cups peeled and chopped apples	Increased fiber
3/4 cup grated carrots	1/2 cup grated carrots	Increased fiber
2 tablespoons chopped pecans	1/2 cup chopped pecans	Reduced fat and calories

Remember—make just one or two changes at a time and note the impact on the recipe.

Beans are very versatile. They take on the flavor of the foods with which they're cooked. Add beans to vegetable soup or meat filling in Mexican foods, or enjoy a meatless meal, such as red beans and rice, a few days each week. Beans do contain carbohydrate, so be sure to count 15 grams of carbohydrate for each 1/2 cup cooked beans.

See Chapter 8 for more information on fiber and tips to increase fiber in your meal plan.

Fiber-Fortified Foods: At a Glance

The nutrition recommendations from the American Diabetes Association encourage individuals with diabetes to eat the same amount of fiber suggested for the general public: about 25 grams of fiber per day for adult women and 38 grams of fiber per day for adult men. In addition, at least half of all the grains you eat should be whole grains. Most Americans are falling far short of these numbers. *Should you include fiber-fortified foods in your meal plan to help you reach these goals?*

Food manufacturers have begun fiber-fortifying foods such as yogurt, cereals, breads, fruit juices, milk, tortillas, baked goods, ice cream, and candies as well as supplement bars and beverages. **This fiber can provide health benefits in one of three ways:**

- **Bulking fibers** (noted on nutrition information labels by names such as carboxymethyl cellulose, methyl-cellulose, or wheat bran) add bulk to the stool and may help reduce constipation while improving digestive health.
- **Viscous fibers** (noted on nutrition information labels by names such as agar, guar gum, or pectin) may help lower blood cholesterol and assist with blood glucose control and weight management efforts.
- **Fermentable fibers** (noted on nutrition information labels by names such as inulin, psyllium, or resistant starch) may result in increased mineral absorption, immune support, and insulin sensitivity.

Most nutrition experts agree that **it's best to get fiber from a wide variety of foods.** Fiber-fortified foods may not provide the vitamins, minerals, and other beneficial nutrients found in naturally high-fiber foods. If you are considering using a fiber-fortified food, read its nutrition information label and ingredient list carefully. Keep in mind, too, that fiber supplements can interfere with the absorption of certain medications and may reduce blood glucose levels, which could require an adjustment in your diabetes medications.

Your RD/RDN or diabetes health-care team can recommend ways to increase the amount of high-fiber foods in your meal plan or help you decide if including fiber-fortified foods in your meal plan is the right choice for you.

Fortifying the Flavor

No matter how healthy the recipe, the most important ingredient is good flavor. Consumer research has shown that flavor is the reason we favor one food over another. It stands to reason that if you're reducing some ingredients—to cut back on fat, sugar, and salt—you may need to fortify the flavor in other ways.

Cook's Notes: 3 Tips to Enrich and Enhance Flavor

1. Use the freshest ingredients you can find when cooking. If you can't buy fresh fruits and vegetables, use frozen versions. Frozen products are generally frozen immediately after picking, so they retain their flavor better than the canned, processed versions of fruits and vegetables. Also, they're lower in sodium.

2. Add herbs to pack a flavor punch.
   - Dry herbs are stronger than fresh; use 1 teaspoon of a dried herb to substitute for 1 tablespoon of the fresh variety.
   - For chilled foods, such as salad dressings and dips, add herbs several hours before serving to allow time for their flavors to blend.

Enhanced Eggnog

A few simple switches take eggnog from simply tasting good, to tasting good *and* being better for you. This version is lower in fat, calories, and sugar, yet enhanced in flavor.

Use this:	Instead of this:	And you get:
1/4 cup egg substitute or two egg whites for each whole egg in the recipe	Whole eggs	Reduced fat and calories
3/4 cup sugar	1 1/2 cups sugar	Reduced sugar and calories
Light whipped topping	Cream	Reduced fat and calories
Rum extract	Liquor	Reduced calories and increased flavor
Low-fat milk	Whole milk	Reduced fat and calories
Ginger, ground cinnamon, nutmeg	Liquor	Reduced calories and increased flavor

Remember—make just one or two changes at a time and note the impact on the recipe.

- When making a hot dish, such as a soup or stew, add herbs toward the end of the cooking time, so their flavor won't disappear.

3. Squeeze citrus on steamed vegetables instead of using butter or over a salad instead of using dressing. The juice from a fresh lemon, lime, or orange can fortify flavor without adding calories.

Good-for-You Foods Should Taste Good, Too

When all is said and done, taste, not health benefits, is the reason most people choose one food over another. However, with the tricks of the trade you've learned in this chapter, you no longer have to decide between a favorite recipe and good blood glucose control. It takes more than good ingredients and good techniques to be a good cook—be willing to experiment and enjoy!

Smart Subs

Even one or two simple recipe changes can improve the nutritional value of your favorite family recipes. Table 9.3 has a few ideas to get you started.

Table 9.3   Smart Recipe Substitutions

If your recipe calls for this:	Substitute this healthier choice:
Bacon	Canadian bacon, turkey bacon, smoked turkey, or lean prosciutto (italian ham)
Beef, ground	Lean ground beef (90% lean or higher), lean ground chicken, or lean ground turkey breast
Bread crumbs, dry	Rolled oats or crushed high-fiber cereal
Bread, white	100% whole-wheat bread
Butter, margarine, shortening, or oil (in baked goods)	Applesauce, puréed pumpkin, puréed sweet potato, mashed bananas, or prune purée (for half of the butter, shortening, or oil). Note: avoid using diet whipped or tub-style margarine in place of regular margarine.
Butter, margarine, shortening, or oil (to prevent sticking)	Cooking spray and/or nonstick pans
Cheddar cheese (1 cup)	Extra-sharp reduced-fat cheddar cheese (1/2 cup)
Chocolate chips (1 cup)	Dark chocolate chips (1/2 cup) or mini chocolate chips (3/4 cup)

(continued on next page)

Table 9.3	Smart Recipe Substitutions *(Continued)*
If your recipe calls for this:	**Substitute this healthier choice:**
Cream, heavy (1 cup)	Heavy cream (1/2 cup) plus fat-free plain yogurt (1/2 cup) OR evaporated skim milk (1 cup)
Cream cheese, full fat	Fat-free or low-fat cream cheese, Neufchâtel, or low-fat cottage cheese puréed until smooth
Egg	2 egg whites or 1/4 cup egg substitute for each whole egg in the recipe
Flour, all-purpose white (1 cup)	White flour (1/2 cup) plus whole-wheat flour (1/2 cup) OR whole-wheat pastry flour (1 cup)
Fruit canned in heavy syrup	Fruit canned in its own juice/water or fresh fruit
Lettuce, iceberg	Arugula, chicory, collard greens, dandelion greens, kale, mustard greens, romaine lettuce, spinach, or watercress
Marinade, oil-based	Wine, balsamic vinegar, fruit juice, or fat-free broth
Mayonnaise	Reduced-calorie mayonnaise-type salad dressing; reduced-calorie, reduced-fat mayonnaise; fat-free plain yogurt or fat-free plain greek yogurt
Meat (as the main ingredient)	Extra vegetables in place of meat on pizzas or in casseroles; beans in soups and stews
Milk, evaporated	Evaporated skim milk
Milk, whole	Reduced-fat or fat-free milk
Pasta, white	Whole-wheat or fiber-enriched pasta
Rice, white	Brown rice, wild rice, bulgur, or pearl barley
Salt	Omit and use extra herbs and spices, citrus juices, rice vinegar, or salt-free seasoning mixes
Seasoning salt (such as garlic, celery, or onion salt)	Herb/spice-only seasonings, such as garlic powder, celery seed, or onion flakes OR use finely chopped herbs or garlic, celery, or onions

(continued on next page)

Table 9.3	Smart Recipe Substitutions *(Continued)*
If your recipe calls for this:	**Substitute this healthier choice:**
Soups, creamed	Fat-free milk-based soups—add mashed potato flakes or puréed carrots to thicken
Sour cream, full fat	Fat-free or low-fat sour cream, plain fat-free or low-fat yogurt or greek yogurt
Soy sauce	Low-sodium soy sauce
Sugar, white or brown	In most baked goods, you can reduce the amount of sugar by one-half; adding vanilla, nutmeg, or cinnamon to the recipe intensifies the sweetness
Syrup	Fresh berries, puréed fruits (such as applesauce), or sugar-free syrup

Next Steps

Modify one favorite family recipe. Try to reduce the fat, sugar, and salt, and increase the fiber and flavor.

What Do I Eat for Dinner?

FOR 45–60 GRAMS OF CARBOHYDRATE*

3 ounces grilled barbecue chicken breast
   on 100% whole-wheat bun
1/4 cup broccoli slaw
Recipe: Not-So-Devilish Eggs (2 egg halves)
1 cup cubed cantaloupe or honeydew

FOR 60–75 GRAMS OF CARBOHYDRATE*

3 ounces grilled barbecue chicken breast
   on 100% whole-wheat bun
1 small (or 1/2 large) piece corn on the cob
1/4 cup broccoli slaw
Recipe: Not-So-Devilish Eggs (2 egg halves)
1 cup cubed cantaloupe or honeydew

*For most women, 45–60 grams of carbohydrate at a meal is a good starting point; for most men, 60–75 grams of carbohydrate per meal is appropriate. Check with your diabetes health-care team to find the amount of carbohydrate that's right for you.

Swift, Simple Tip

- Use your microwave to quick-cook corn on the cob in its own natural moisture. Leaving the husks and silk intact, place ears of corn on a dampened paper towel on a microwave-safe plate. Turn ears over and rearrange after half of the cooking time has passed.

  Cooking Timetable:
  - 1 ear: 1 1/2 minutes
  - 2 ears: 3–4 minutes
  - 3 ears: 5–6 minutes
  - 4 ears: 7–8 minutes
  - 6 ears: 8–9 minutes

  When ears are hot to the touch, carefully remove from microwave and wrap in a kitchen towel or foil. Let stand at least 5 minutes. Remove husks and silk (which is easier than when corn is cold) and serve. Season the corn with spices—such as basil, garlic, rosemary, sage, or thyme—to enhance the flavor without adding extra calories.

- If you're short on time, rather than slicing and chopping the vegetables for broccoli slaw yourself, pick up a bag of prepared broccoli slaw, which contains ready-to-mix broccoli, carrots, and red cabbage.

NOT-SO-DEVILISH EGGS

SERVES: 8

SERVING SIZE: 2 egg halves

PREPARATION TIME: 45 minutes

COOKING TIME: Included in prep time

INGREDIENTS

8 large eggs

1/4 cup water

1/4 cup cider vinegar

1 tablespoon sugar

1/4 cup finely chopped red onion

2 tablespoons fat-free plain greek yogurt

2 tablespoons fat-free mayonnaise

2 teaspoons dijon mustard

1/2 teaspoon creamy horseradish

1/4 teaspoon freshly ground black pepper

2 tablespoons finely chopped chives

Recipe Tip

- Rather than hard boiling eggs the day of purchase, boil eggs that you've had in the refrigerator for 7–10 days for easier and quicker peeling. After cooking, let the eggs rest in an ice bath; bringing the temperature down quickly means the papery membrane is more likely to stick to the shell rather than the egg.

1. Hard boil the eggs: Place eggs in a saucepan large enough to hold them in a single layer and cover with 1–2 inches of cold water. Heat over high heat just to boiling. Remove from burner. Cover pan. Let eggs stand in hot water for about 12 minutes. Drain immediately, then cool eggs completely in a bowl of ice water. Once cooled, drain the water from the eggs.

2. While eggs are cooking, combine 1/4 cup water, cider vinegar, and sugar in a medium, microwave-safe bowl. Microwave on high 2 minutes or until boiling. Stir in red onion. Let stand at room temperature 15 minutes. Drain.

3. Combine yogurt, mayonnaise, mustard, horseradish, and pepper in a medium bowl, stirring well to combine.

4. Peel eggs and discard shells. Slice eggs in half lengthwise and remove and reserve yolks. Add 6 yolks to yogurt mixture; reserving remaining yolks for another use. Mash yogurt/yolk mixture with a fork until very smooth. Stir in 2 tablespoons of red onion. Spoon mixture into egg white halves (about 1 tablespoon in each half). Garnish egg halves with remaining red onion and chives.

CHOICES/EXCHANGES

1 Medium-Fat Protein

BASIC NUTRITIONAL VALUES

Calories	70	**Potassium**	90 mg
Calories from Fat	30	**Total Carbohydrate**	3 g
Total Fat	3.5 g	Dietary Fiber	0 g
Saturated Fat	1.2 g	Sugars	2 g
Trans Fat	0.0 g	**Protein**	6 g
Cholesterol	135 mg	**Phosphorus**	65 mg
Sodium	125 mg		

Food for Thought

- **Your favorite recipes can be "made over"** to decrease the fat, sugar, and salt content and increase the fiber and flavor.
- **Review each ingredient in your recipe.** What is its function? Can the ingredient be changed without ruining the recipe?
- **Think of your kitchen as a cooking "lab."** Don't be afraid to experiment and make modifications. Limit your changes to only one or two ingredients at a time so you can determine whether the substitutions work.

CHAPTER 10

S pecial occasions are an important part of life—be it holiday gatherings, parties, a toast to an accomplishment, or a trip. Each brings unique eating opportunities and challenges and this chapter equips you with a multitude of practical strategies and tips to successfully navigate a variety of situations, including:

- Social gatherings
- Alcohol consumption
- Travel

Parties and Holidays: Let the Fun Begin!

Since diabetes entered your life, have you ever felt like skipping out on holiday feasts, family gatherings, birthday parties, or any other kind of party because of the potential eating challenges you'll face? Missing out on all of those celebrations certainly is not necessary. In fact, with a few strategies in place, you can make it through almost any social situation without sabotaging your diabetes control.

Social Gathering Strategy #1: Share and Share Alike

If you are concerned that the food at a party or holiday meal will be swimming in fat and chock-full of carbohydrate and calories, then offer to bring a healthier dish to share that suits your tastes and nutrition needs. That way you'll know there's at least one item you can munch on without worry. And your host is likely to appreciate having an addition to the party spread

An Awesome, Easy Vegetable Platter

Looking for a healthy dish to bring to the next social gathering you attend? Consider a vegetable platter! Rather than compartmentalizing each type of vegetable, jam everything possible onto a platter, using a bit of care to make sure that colors are spaced out and that all the vegetables are showing their best side. Scatter two or three small bowls of flavored hummus throughout for dunking the vegetables. Here are some vegetable options you may want to include:

For a taste twist, try:	The oldies, but goodies:
Asparagus of different colors (lightly steamed) Baby corn Broccoli rabe or broccolini (lightly steamed) Cherry or grape tomatoes Edamame (soybeans in the pod) Jicama Red, green, and yellow bell pepper strips Sugar snap peas Zucchini or summer squash strips	Broccoli florets Cauliflower florets Celery sticks Baby carrots Cucumber sticks

without having to prepare it. The recipes for Pear Dessert "Nachos" and Individual Bite-Size S'mores at the end of this chapter are simple, tasty, and fun desserts you might consider taking to share at the next social gathering.

Social Gathering Strategy #2: Take a Cruise (Along the Party Spread, That Is!)

Before filling a plate, cruise the holiday buffet or party spread and decide which foods you really want and what portion of each best fits your carbohydrate goals. Ask yourself,

"*Is it worth the carbohydrate or calories?*" If the answer is "no," then pass it by. If the answer is "yes," then decide what portion fits your carbohydrate budget and add it to your plate.

Social Gathering Strategy #3: Fill Half of Your Plate with Veggies

Rather than packing your plate with high-calorie appetizers, fill at least half of your plate with raw veggies. (If you bring a vegetable platter, then you've got this covered.) Raw vegetables will keep you munching and fill you up with minimal carbohydrate and calorie cost, leaving room in your carbohydrate "budget" to sample some special foods.

Social Gathering Strategy #4: Plan and Incorporate, Rather Than Add On

Have you ever tried to trick yourself into believing that "just a little bit" of a treat won't affect your blood glucose? The reality is, that strategy doesn't work out so well, especially when carbohydrate foods are involved. So whether it's a cocktail party, birthday party, holiday dinner, or the biggest candy day of the year (Halloween), keep tabs on your portions and the associated amount of carbohydrate you've consumed so you can work in a tasty treat as *part of your carbohydrate count* for the eating occasion. By planning and incorporating the treat or special food, rather than simply adding it onto your meal plan, you can truly have your cake (or candy) and eat it, too—without sacrificing blood glucose control!

Social Gathering Strategy #5: Think Before You Drink

Decide your alcoholic drink limit before any special occasion. At the big event, start with a nonalcoholic beverage to satisfy your thirst and then savor one alcoholic beverage by slowly sipping. If you choose to have more than one alcoholic drink, make the drink in between nonalcoholic. That way, you'll consume less alcohol and give your body time to process the alcohol you've already had.

It's important to know that alcohol consumption may place you at increased risk for delayed hypoglycemia, especially if you take

It's Not Too Spooky!

When the craving for a sweet treat strikes, you can satisfy your sweet tooth with these treats for about 15 grams of carbohydrate each:

- 8 pieces of candy corn
- 3 Hershey's miniature candy bars
- 6 jelly beans
- 1 fun-size Milky Way bar
- 3 red and white peppermint or cinnamon hard candies
- 1 fun-size Twix
- 10 Whoppers (1 small pouch)

Of course we're not advocating that you eat these, but if you do choose to eat a sweet treat, we want you to know the best way to do so.

How Much Alcohol Is Too Much?

If you choose to drink alcohol, the American Diabetes Association recommends no more than one alcoholic drink per day for women and no more than two per day for men.

off a few extra calories. We've run across many patients over the years who like to crank up their favorite music and just dance it out at home.

If alcohol and dancing are part of your party scene, keep an even closer watch on your blood glucose because the combination of alcohol and physical activity may leave you with lower blood glucose than expected.

insulin or other diabetes medications that can cause hypoglycemia. (Unsure about any diabetes medications you're taking? Ask your pharmacist.) More information about alcohol follows later in this chapter.

Social Gathering Strategy #6: Dance the Night Away

To help head off unwanted weight gain and keep your blood glucose in the target range, make sure to keep moving and get some physical activity each day. While raking leaves, shoveling snow, and walking the dog all count, dancing is also fantastic physical activity and it's fun at parties! So hit the dance floor when possible and work

Social Gathering Strategy #7: Always Be Prepared

When heading out the door to the festivities, remember to take:

- Any diabetes medicines you'll need
- Your meter and testing supplies
- A quick-acting carbohydrate source, such as glucose tablets (especially if you take glucose-lowering medicines and are planning to have a drink or two)

If you're not certain what foods will be available or when they'll be served, stash a carbohydrate snack or two in your pocket or bag, just in case your blood glucose starts to fall.

Are the Calories Worth It?

Are the party foods worth the amount of activity necessary to burn off the extra calories?

A 150-pound woman would have to:

- Walk about 30 minutes at 3 miles per hour to burn off one 12-ounce light beer
- Dance energetically for about 40 minutes to burn off one slice of apple pie
- Cycle for about 10 minutes to burn off a 1-ounce cube of cheese

3 Snacks to Pack and Go

- Small box of raisins
- Four-pack of cheese crackers or peanut butter crackers
- Chewy granola bar

Have Fun!

Eat a small snack to curb your appetite before you head out to the festivities. That way, you can focus on fun and fellowship with friends and family, rather than being sidetracked by your appetite.

Small, Smart Pre-Party Snacks

- Small handful of walnuts or almonds
- Single-serve cup of greek yogurt
- One stick of string cheese

Avoid the "Seasonal Seven"!

Want to keep yourself honest during the holidays and avoid the seasonal 7-pound weight gain?

Wear your most form-fitting pants or jeans frequently during the season. If they start to get tight, it's definitely time to make changes to your habits.

Alcohol and Diabetes: The Mixer

Whether it's a beer with friends after work, a glass of wine at a dinner party, or a champagne toast on New Year's Eve, alcoholic beverages are frequently part of today's social life. So, you may be wondering how alcohol and diabetes mix. If you like to enjoy an occasional alcoholic beverage, the good news is that you most likely can continue to do so (unless some of your medications or other health conditions prevent it). Moderation is key. As noted earlier in this chapter, the American Diabetes Association recommends no more than one alcoholic drink per day for women and no more than two per day for men.

What Is One Drink?

One alcoholic drink has about 100 calories and is equal to:

- 12 ounces of beer
- 5 ounces of dry red or white wine
- 5 ounces of champagne
- 1 1/2 ounces of distilled spirits
- 3 1/2 ounces of dessert wine

3 Considerations If You Choose to Sip an Occasional Alcoholic Beverage:

- Calories
- Carbohydrate
- Potential increased risk for hypoglycemia

> ## Take a Pass
>
> Avoid drinking alcoholic beverages if you:
>
> - Take medicines or have a medical history that suggests you should avoid alcohol use
> - Are pregnant or trying to become pregnant
> - Have liver disease, pancreatitis, advanced neuropathy, or high triglycerides
> - Have a history of alcohol abuse or dependence
> - Are going to be driving

Calories Count

Alcohol has no real nutritional value, but you do need to factor in the calories, especially if you are trying to lose weight. (See the "What Is One Drink?" box for the calorie content of common alcoholic beverages.) Check out the calories in the three common mixed drinks listed below. These are 4-ounce portions, so you may need to double or triple the calories and carbohydrate amounts given depending on the size of the beverage you are served.

- **4-ounce margarita**—185 calories and 16 grams of carbohydrate
- **4-ounce cosmopolitan**—213 calories and 13 grams of carbohydrate
- **4-ounce daiquiri**—224 calories and 9 grams of carbohydrate

Consider as well that alcohol consumption reduces inhibitions and self-control, which may lead to munching down more calories and carbohydrate than planned.

Carbohydrate Can Be a Concern

Distilled Spirits and Mixed Drinks

When it comes to carbohydrate, straight distilled spirits (including gin, rum, tequila, vodka, and whiskey) do not have any carbohydrate and thus do not directly affect blood glucose levels. However, be aware of the carbohydrate in any mixers because those can impact your blood glucose. For instance, a 4-ounce mojito contains 16 grams of carbohydrate.

Wine and Champagne

Dry wines and champagne have minimal carbohydrate, though sweet dessert wines are a different story. For sweet dessert wines, you'll have to count the equivalent of 1 carbohydrate choice (15 grams of carbohydrate) for a 5-ounce glass.

Beer

Light beers (<4.5% alcohol by volume) and low-carbohydrate beers are lower in

> ## Alcohol Strategy #1
>
> To control carbohydrate and calories from alcoholic beverages, choose light or low-carbohydrate beer, dry white or red wine, champagne, or "skinny" mixed drinks (those with low-calorie/carbohydrate mixers). Carbohydrate-free mixers include diet sodas, diet tonic water, and club soda.

carbohydrate than regular or dark beers. Per 12-ounce serving, light beers are equivalent to 1/2 carbohydrate choice (about 7.5 grams of carbohydrate), while regular beer is one carbohydrate choice (15 grams of carbohydrate) and dark beers are 1–1 1/2 carbohydrate choices.

High or Low: Which Way Will the Blood Glucose Go?

As mentioned earlier in this chapter, moderate alcohol consumption generally has minimal effect on blood glucose in people with diabetes (with the exception of carbohydrate-rich beverages). However, excessive amounts of alcohol (three or more drinks per day) on a consistent basis may cause high blood glucose.

With all that said, it's important to be aware that delayed hypoglycemia is a possibility when people with diabetes drink alcohol, especially for those taking insulin or other diabetes medications that can cause hypoglycemia. Why? Very simply put, one of your liver's jobs is to put out glucose to help maintain your blood glucose levels, but when you drink alcohol, the liver switches over to processing the alcohol and glucose output is decreased. As a result, blood glucose levels may drop—sometimes too low.

An Ounce of Prevention

Think before you drink. Here are a few tips to help you drink smart:

- **Have a plan.** Discuss with your health-care team how to safely fit alcohol into your diabetes plan.
- **Stay on target.** Drink alcohol only if your blood glucose levels are in your target range most of the time.
- **If low, then "no go."** Do not drink alcohol if you have low blood glucose.
- **Know your limits.** Limit alcohol to no more than one drink per day if you're a woman and two drinks per day or fewer if you're a man.
- **Wear your medical ID.** Make sure you wear a medical identification when drinking because symptoms of hypoglycemia can be confused with intoxication.

Alcohol Strategy #2

To reduce the risk of low blood glucose, particularly if you take insulin or other glucose-lowering medications, never drink alcohol on an empty stomach. Always eat a food that has carbohydrate when drinking an alcoholic beverage.

Alcohol Strategy #3

To find out how alcohol affects you, keep a close watch on your blood glucose levels by checking more frequently than usual. *When should you check your blood glucose?*

While you're drinking alcohol:

- If your blood glucose approaches 70 mg/dL or below and it's not mealtime, eat a 15–30-gram carbohydrate snack.

One to two hours after drinking alcohol:

- If, during waking hours, your blood glucose approaches 70 mg/dL or below and it's not mealtime, eat a 15–30-gram carbohydrate snack.

Before going to bed:

- If you typically eat a bedtime snack, you should still eat it.
- If you don't typically eat a bedtime snack, but you take diabetes medications and your blood glucose is <100 mg/dL at bedtime, then eat a 15–30-gram carbohydrate snack.

During the night after drinking alcoholic beverages:

- Set an alarm to wake you up. If a middle-of-the-night blood glucose check is <100 mg/dL, eat a 15–30-gram carbohydrate snack. Put a snack that does not require refrigeration by your bed before going to sleep so you don't have to get up to get it if you need it. Easy snack ideas for this purpose include peanut butter crackers or a granola bar.

Most importantly, consult with your diabetes health-care team about how to personalize these recommendations to suit you.

What Are You Drinking?

Lower carbohydrate content	Higher carbohydrate content
Light or low-carbohydrate beer	Sweet wine
Dry white or red wine	Wine coolers
Dry champagne	Liqueurs
Distilled liquors, straight (such as bourbon, gin, rum, scotch, vodka)	Mixed drinks with sweet, sugar-containing mixers (such as daiquiris, margaritas, and mojitos)

Alcohol Alternatives

Looking for a lower-alcohol alternative?

- Try a wine spritzer. Mix two parts wine with one part club soda.

Looking for nonalcoholic alternatives?

- Club soda, sparkling water, or water with a twist of lemon, lime, or orange
- Diet tonic water with a twist of lime
- Nonalcoholic beer
- "Virgin" cocktails

3 More Tips to Sip By

- **Dilute your drink.** Dilute drinks with club soda, seltzer, or ice to make them last longer.
- **Pick your party pals wisely.** Alcohol can make it harder to realize that your blood glucose is low because the symptoms of intoxication resemble those of hypoglycemia. Alcohol may impair your thought processes, too. So make sure you have a pal around who knows you have diabetes and knows how to treat hypoglycemia.
- **Check, check, and check.** Keep your blood glucose monitor handy and check your blood glucose frequently to head off hypoglycemia.

Have Diabetes, Will Travel

Diabetes is your constant companion, but traveling can be a smooth ride if you do a little planning ahead! Whether your itinerary includes a short road trip, cruising to an exotic port, or flying to the far corners of the earth, now's the time to draft a plan to keep you in the best possible state of health (and mind) before leaving and to help you travel and eat smart once you depart.

5 Tips to Eat Smart While Traveling

Chances are before developing diabetes you occasionally ran into some eating challenges when traveling, whether it was finding something other than a fast-food burger on the road or something other than peanuts or pretzels on an airplane. Now that diabetes is on the scene, having a plan in place to deal with travel-related eating challenges is even more important. The following five tips will help you eat smart and manage your diabetes wherever you are!

Travel Tip #1: Do some investigative work. If you are traveling on a plane or train, check when you make the reservations to see if a meal, snack, or beverage will be offered. Before your travels begin, see what food establishments and markets will be close at hand both during your travels and once you reach your destination. Err on the side of caution and don't count on foods and beverages always being readily available; have a stash with you. (See the list of "20 Travel-Friendly Foods," which follows, for some ideas.) And because traveling and eating out typically go hand in hand, put the tips discussed in Chapter 6 to the test during your trip.

Travel Tip #2: Go local. When trying out local cuisine, one of the most important tips is portion control. Too much carbohydrate translates into higher blood glucose levels. If you have an adventurous palate, but are uncertain of the carbohydrate content of local foods, make your best estimate as to the portion that meets your carbohydrate needs, and then check your blood glucose 1 1/2–2 hours after eating to see how the food affected you. If your blood glucose is out of your target range, take a walk or do some type of physical activity to help lower your blood glucose. If you take rapid-acting insulin based on blood glucose values, then make appropriate adjustments as advised by your diabetes health-care team. Talk in advance with your diabetes health-care team about how to handle this type of situation before you depart for your trip. Learn from the situation so you'll know what to expect if you choose to eat the food again.

Travel Tip #3: Ask and you shall receive. Ask hotels for a small refrigerator and/or microwave in your room. You can keep a few snacks or beverages chilled or prepare instant oats or a cup of soup.

Travel Tip #4: Ask restaurants for what you need. For instance, that might be an egg and toast rather than pastries for breakfast.

Travel Tip #5: Take a test drive. Test your travel plan by taking a short weekend road trip (before tackling a 2-week trek across the globe, for example) to master the eating and diabetes challenges that accompany travel.

20 Travel-Friendly Foods

Travel with plenty of ready-to-eat, portable snacks in case of meal delays or food unavailability. Here are a few examples:

1. Individual portions of peanut butter and pretzel sticks
2. Peanut butter sandwich (natural peanut butter on whole-grain bread)
3. Whole-grain crackers or a bagel with peanut butter or another nut butter
4. Vacuum-packed tuna or salmon and crackers
5. Reduced-sodium jerky
6. Individual portion packs or zip-top bags of almonds, pistachios, peanuts, soy nuts, or roasted pumpkin seeds
7. Small packs or zip-top bags filled with high-fiber cereal
8. Homemade or store-bought trail mix in zip-top bags
9. Fresh fruit (apples, small bananas, clementines, zip-top bags of grapes)
10. Single-serving containers of applesauce or fruit packed in juice
11. Small boxes of raisins
12. Dried fruit in zip-top bags
13. Raw vegetables in zip-top bags or individual portion packs (baby carrots, celery sticks, grape tomatoes)
14. Low-fat popcorn in a zip-top bag
15. Cereal or granola bars (choose those with 5 grams of fiber or more per serving)
16. Protein bars (choose those that fit within your carbohydrate goals with minimal to no added sugar)
17. Single-serving beverages (juice boxes, bottled water, boxed milk, or canned tomato juice or vegetable juice)
18. Single-serving yogurt cups
19. Cheese and crackers (whole-grain crackers with low-fat string cheese)
20. Individually wrapped reduced-fat cheeses

To prevent food spoilage, don't keep perishable foods at room temperature for longer than 2 hours total. Use a small, soft-sided cooler with freezer packs for transporting perishable foods.

10 Tips to Travel Smart with Diabetes

Tip #1: Identify yourself. Wear your medical identification (bracelet, necklace, etc.) that says you have diabetes and notes if you take insulin. Carry a note from your doctor explaining your diabetes supplies, medicines, devices, and any allergies, along with the information for an emergency contact. Remember to carry your medical insurance card (and travel medical coverage if out of the country). Also carry a list of the members of your health-care team and their contact information just in case the need to reach them arises.

Tip #2: Over-pack your medicines and diabetes supplies. You never know when you'll run into a travel delay, so pack double the amount of medicine and supplies you think you'll need. Gone for 5 days? Pack 10 days' worth.

Tip #3: Ease through airports. Before air travel, you can always check with the Transportation Security Administration (TSA) for the latest travel updates and to learn about current screening policies (visit www.tsa.gov). Tell the TSA agents that you have diabetes.

Tip #4: Keep your medicines and supplies close. Keep them close at hand by packing them in your carry-on bag to prevent damage and avoid losing them at the airport. Insulin, other medications, and testing supplies are temperature-sensitive so avoid storing them in the trunk, glove compartment, back window of the car, or in a checked bag at the airport. Keep them in the original packaging so there's no question along the way as to what they are and who they belong to. And don't worry about the liquid carry-on limit on planes; the TSA allows you to exceed those limits for diabetes medications and supplies.

Tip #5: Carry snacks and treatment for low blood glucose. Food access is often unpredictable with travel, so carry portable snacks that won't spoil to head off hunger or treat low blood glucose (if you are at risk for that). A number of options are shared in the list of "20 Travel-Friendly Foods" on page 187. Also stash glucose tablets, gels, or hard candy in your pocket or carry-on bag for easy access.

Tip #6: Do tell. If you are traveling alone, let the flight attendant or conductor know that you have diabetes, just in case you have a problem or require assistance.

Tip #7: Favor your feet. Wear well-fitting, comfortable shoes and socks at all times. Consider wearing light compression stockings if on a long flight or road trip, or if your feet swell otherwise. Check your feet frequently for blisters, cuts, or sores—especially after long walks.

Tip #8: Prepare for a health emergency. Keep a small first aid kit handy. Prior to travel, check out local doctors in the area surrounding your destination who treat diabetes (and who speak English, if traveling abroad).

Tip #9: Keep a closer check on blood glucose. New foods, increased activity, and different time zones can throw your blood glucose off, so test more frequently, especially before and after meals.

Tip #10: The best defense is a good offense. First and foremost, when traveling, try to stay as close to your usual food and medication schedule as possible. Granted, that may be easier said than done, particularly when factoring in flight delays, road construction, traffic jams, and time zone changes. If you take

> ## Did You Know That Airplane Air Dehydrates You?
>
> Dehydration can result in fatigue, feeling thirsty, and worsening sinus problems, and can contribute to swollen feet/ankles and constipation.
>
> - **TIP:** Since beverage service is limited on many flights, allow time to buy one or two bottles of water after passing through airport security and sip the water throughout your flight. Aim to down 8 ounces for every hour of the flight.
> - **TIP:** Skip alcoholic beverages because they can further dehydrate you.

insulin and will be crossing time zones, talk with your health-care team before your trip so they can help you plan the timing of your insulin injections and meals. Keep in mind that westward travel means a longer day (so possibly more insulin will be needed), and eastward travel means a shorter day (so possibly less insulin will be needed). By planning for the unexpected, you'll be ready when any travel-related eating or medication challenges come your way. After all, the best defense is a good offense.

10 Additional Travel Tips for Going Abroad

No one likes to think about the possibility of needing medical care while on a trip. However, advance planning can bring peace of mind when traveling outside the country and help you be prepared should a health event arise.

Here are a few tips* to help you prepare for international travel:

1. Get appropriate immunizations.
2. One month before you leave, visit your health-care team for a checkup.
3. Make plans for temporary health insurance coverage if your plan is not effective outside the U.S.
4. Write down a few diabetes-related phrases in the language of the country you're visiting, such as, "I have diabetes," "I need sugar," or "Where is the hospital?"
5. Wear diabetes identification in the languages of the countries you're visiting.
6. Use bottled water to drink and brush your teeth.
7. Avoid raw fruits and vegetables.
8. Skip beverages with ice.
9. Eat only dairy products that are pasteurized.
10. Always carry snacks with you.

---

*This is not an all-inclusive list.

Next Steps

List two eating strategies you can put into practice at your next social or holiday gathering.

1. _____
2. _____

If you drink alcohol, identify one nonalcoholic beverage that you would be willing to drink at your next event to help minimize alcohol consumption.

1. _____

List two eating strategies or tips you will put into practice on your next trip.

1. _____
2. _____

What Do I Eat for Dinner?

HOLIDAY MEAL FOR 45–60 GRAMS OF CARBOHYDRATE*

3 ounces turkey breast
2 tablespoons turkey gravy
1/2 cup mashed potatoes OR 1/3 cup stuffing
1/2 cup green beans
3 tablespoons whole-berry cranberry sauce
Recipe: Pear Dessert "Nachos" (1 serving)
 OR 2 Individual Bite-Size S'mores

HOLIDAY MEAL FOR 60–75 GRAMS OF CARBOHYDRATE*

3 ounces turkey breast
2 tablespoons turkey gravy
1/2 cup mashed potatoes
1/3 cup stuffing
1/2 cup green beans
3 tablespoons whole-berry cranberry sauce
Recipe: Pear Dessert "Nachos" (1 serving)
 OR 2 Individual Bite-Size S'mores

*For most women, 45–60 grams of carbohydrate at a meal is a good starting point; for most men, 60–75 grams of carbohydrate per meal is appropriate. Check with your diabetes health-care team to find the amount of carbohydrate that's right for you.

Swift, Simple Tips

- Buy a roasted turkey from the local supermarket deli.
- Buy microwave-in-the-bag green beans.

PEAR DESSERT "NACHOS"

SERVES: 3

SERVING SIZE: 3 3/4 ounces (1/3rd recipe)

PREPARATION TIME: 10 minutes

COOKING TIME: 0 minutes

INGREDIENTS

1 (9-ounce) pear, slightly firm and not overly ripe (alternatively, a red or green apple can be used—red if you prefer sweet; green if you prefer tart)

1/4 large lemon or 1/2 small lemon

1 tablespoon sliced almonds (sliced is important in this recipe to get adequate coverage of the nachos)

1 tablespoon sweetened flaked coconut

1 tablespoon all-natural almond butter (any other nut butter can be used)

2 teaspoons mini chocolate chips

2 tablespoons reduced-sugar dried cranberries

1/8 teaspoon ground cinnamon

Recipe Tips

- Almond butter and other nut butters are generally found in grocery stores on the shelf alongside peanut butter.
- While best if served soon after preparation, leftovers are still tasty the next day. The lemon juice keeps the pear (or apple) slices from browning.

1. Quarter and core the pear, then thinly slice it and place in a large bowl. Squeeze juice from lemon evenly over pear slices and toss to coat well. (This step is essential to keep the pear from browning, especially if made ahead.) Arrange pear slices in a single layer on a 10-inch plate. Set aside.

2. Place almonds and coconut on a small tray or piece of aluminum foil. Lightly toast in toaster oven (or broil on low, 3–4 inches from broiler) about 3–4 minutes, or until lightly golden.

3. Meanwhile place almond butter in a small, microwave-safe container and warm until it becomes liquid (about 30–40 seconds if refrigerated; less if at room temperature). Stir well. Using a small spoon, drizzle or gently shake almond butter evenly over pear slices.

4. Sprinkle slices evenly with mini chocolate chips, toasted almonds, toasted coconut, and cranberries. Sprinkle lightly with cinnamon. Best if served soon after preparation.

CHOICES/EXCHANGES	BASIC NUTRITIONAL VALUES			
1 Carbohydrate, 1 Fat	**Calories**	110	**Potassium**	125 mg
	Calories from Fat	50	**Total Carbohydrate**	16 g
	Total Fat	6.0 g	Dietary Fiber	4 g
	Saturated Fat	1.5 g	Sugars	9 g
	Trans Fat	0.0 g	**Protein**	2 g
	Cholesterol	0 mg	**Phosphorus**	45 mg
	Sodium	5 mg		

INDIVIDUAL BITE-SIZE S'MORES

SERVES: 1

SERVING SIZE: 1 s'more

PREPARATION TIME: 2 minutes

COOKING TIME: 4 minutes

INGREDIENTS

1/4 teaspoon almond butter (or any other nut butter)

1 vanilla wafer

1 mini marshmallow

1 dark chocolate kiss-type candy, unwrapped (milk chocolate or other kiss-type candy can be used)

1. Preheat oven or toaster oven to 350°F.
2. Spread almond butter on top of vanilla wafer. Place marshmallow in center and gently push down into the almond butter. Place on baking tray and bake 4 minutes, or until marshmallow starts to turn light golden.
3. Remove from oven and immediately top with kiss candy, pushing it gently into the marshmallow. Best when eaten warm.

Recipe Tips

- The perfect sweet bite, this bite-size dessert is a hit at gatherings and parties at only 6 grams of carbohydrate each!
- Multiply the recipe to make as many as you need.

CHOICES/EXCHANGES
1/2 Carbohydrate, 1/2 Fat

BASIC NUTRITIONAL VALUES

Calories	50	**Potassium**	30 mg
Calories from Fat	20	**Total Carbohydrate**	6 g
Total Fat	2.5 g	Dietary Fiber	0 g
Saturated Fat	0.9 g	Sugars	4 g
Trans Fat	0.0 g	**Protein**	1 g
Cholesterol	5 mg	**Phosphorus**	20 mg
Sodium	15 mg		

Food for Thought

- **Planning ahead and making intentional choices** at social gatherings is essential to managing blood glucose and weight.
- **Limit alcoholic beverages** to no more than one alcoholic drink per day if you are a woman and no more than two per day if you are a man.
- **When traveling, try to stay as close to your usual food and medication schedule as possible.** And keep plenty of travel-friendly snacks on hand.

You may have picked up this book expecting that it would tell you exactly what to eat every day for the rest of your life with diabetes. However, in addition to the specific advice you've received on what to eat, you've also learned about a variety of aspects of diabetes nutrition, so you have the valuable information you need to make healthier choices on your own. In fact, concrete nutrition advice is exactly what you need to survive those first overwhelming days with type 2 diabetes. You've come a long way and, hopefully, you are now more confident when it comes to eating with type 2 diabetes—confident enough that you are able to transition from being *told* what to eat to successfully *making your own decisions* about a wide variety of foods. That's exactly where you are right now—ready to live your life with diabetes with the help of a meal plan that works for you and meets your individual needs.

Meet the Challenge

As you have learned, diabetes isn't like the majority of medical conditions. A simple pill, procedure, or surgery won't just take care of it or make it go away. Although you do have the resources of your diabetes health-care team at your disposal, ultimately you are the one making the daily decisions that affect your health and well-being. Will you make the time for breakfast or skip it? Will you snack on a piece of fresh fruit or a handful of gummy bears? Gaining the experience you need to make the right decisions will undoubtedly be a challenge. Successful diabetes management requires that you not only have knowledge, but also the control, resources, and experience to make the best decisions for your health.

When you face the challenge of maintaining good diabetes control through better nutrition, you must consider your goals as well as strategies and targets. As you learned in the very first chapter of this book, a general goal, such as "I want to lose weight," is not going to be easy to achieve unless you consider strategies that will work for you, such as "I'll get more exercise" or "I'll eat smaller portions." An even greater challenge is to reach for a more specific target—for example, "I'll change from whole milk to fat-free milk" or "I'll have a side salad instead of french fries when I eat fast food." Setting more specific goals and targets that work with your particular lifestyle will be easier for you to reach and will, in turn, give you the confidence you'll need to meet the challenges ahead.

Bottom line? The changes you've made in your meal plan are for life. If you make healthy choices most of the time, it's OK to occasionally eat something that may not be the best for your body. Your body can recover easily from an occasional lapse. Learn from your slip-up and move on!

Are You "Cheating" Yourself?

Have you ever felt guilty because you ate a cupcake, skipped a workout, or couldn't resist the lure of late-night snacking? People often use the word "cheat" to express the shame they feel after making a decision they wish they hadn't. If you find that you're beating yourself up with negative self-talk, here are three things to keep in mind:

1. **The fact that you made a poor eating decision is not as important as what you're going to do about it now.** Don't let an unhealthy choice be an excuse to give up on your meal plan.
2. **Think about why you made the choice that you did.** Were you feeling stressed? Did you let yourself get too hungry? Learn from this situation and plan for what you'll do when you find yourself there again in the future. Next time, maybe you'll treat yourself to a stress-relieving bubble bath instead of grabbing the nearest chocolate bar.
3. **You're setting yourself up for failure if you expect perfection.** Potato chips and pecan pie will always be around. Make peace with that fact and work with your registered dietitian/registered dietitian nutritionist (RD/RDN) to find out how to enjoy those special foods in a healthier way.

Continue to Learn All You Can

A wise man once said, "Experience is a hard teacher. She gives the test first, then the lesson afterward." So it is with life with diabetes. You will find that you gain much by learning from each situation you face. What worked when you were faced with a party buffet? What will you do differently the next time you're traveling?

You've already learned a vast amount about nutrition for type 2 diabetes. With this guide, you have accomplished specific tasks that have set you on the right path for managing your diabetes meal plan on your own.

The "Next Steps" at the end of each chapter of this book have enabled you to do the following:

- Set three S.M.A.R.T. goals for improving your diabetes nutrition and prioritize them.
- Choose your highest-priority nutrition goal, and list three changes you can make today to help you move toward accomplishing it.
- Contact an RD/RDN or certified diabetes educator. Schedule an appointment, and prepare for it by gathering information, such as a list of favorite foods and the carbohydrate counts of portions you typically eat.
- Play with your food by pulling out your measuring cups, spoons, and a food scale to learn more about portion sizes and what you actually eat.
- Put your label-reading skills to the test. Search your pantry shelves to find the carbohydrate counts of foods you have on hand.
- Plan menus for three dinners to serve in the near future and buy the foods to prepare them.
- Identify foods that fit the suggested carbohydrate goals for three meals at your favorite fast-food or quick-service dining venues.
- List two changes that will enable you to fit your favorite fast-food meals into your diabetes nutrition plan.
- Learn more about how eating out affects your blood glucose by checking it 1 1/2–2 hours after the meal. If blood glucose was not on target, rethink your portion sizes and carbohydrate estimates.
- List three snacks you could eat at home and three snacks you might eat on-the-go that meet your taste and nutrition needs.
- Keep a record of everything you eat and drink for 3–4 days. Take inventory of whether you could switch out some foods to improve your fat quality, trim sodium, and boost your fiber.
- Check the portion sizes of your meat servings. Are they the size of the palm of your hand?
- Modify one favorite family recipe. Try to reduce the fat, sugar, and salt,

and increase the fiber and flavor as appropriate.

- List two eating strategies you can put into practice at your next social or holiday gathering.
- If you drink alcohol, identify one non-alcoholic beverage that you will drink at your next event to help minimize alcohol consumption.
- List two eating strategies or tips you will put into practice on your next trip.
- Remember to savor the joy of eating!

You also have a collection of quick, healthy recipes and menus to use every day.

What an impressive list of accomplishments! Each of them took you one step further along the path toward being able to manage your diabetes meal plan on your own. *But the learning doesn't stop here.*

When you put down this book, you might be surprised to suddenly notice the vast amount of available information about diabetes and nutrition. After all, there are over 29 million Americans who have diabetes and who are searching for answers. Some of the advice you receive about diabetes will be given by well-meaning family members and friends. Other information might come from the popular press or your own searches on the Internet. How do you sort out the helpful advice from the old wives' tales, particularly in today's online, electronic environment?

Internet Insight: Reliable Diabetes and Healthy-Eating Information

A seemingly endless amount of diabetes information is available on the Internet. The problem is figuring out whether this information is safe and reliable. Be skeptical. Things that sound too good to be true often are. To find the best health resources, ask these questions:

- Who sponsors the website you are browsing? Look for an "About Us" page. Are ads/sponsored content clearly labeled?
- What are the credentials of those who provide information for the site? Does the site have an editorial board?
- When was the site last updated? Health information is constantly changing.
- What does your diabetes health-care team think about the information you've found? Information you find on a website does not replace your health-care team's advice.

One experience with unreliable Internet information:

Many times throughout our years in practice, we've had patients come in voicing the belief that **"white foods are bad"** based on a story they read on the Internet. The belief that people with diabetes should avoid all white foods is false. The idea of avoiding anything white seems to have blossomed out of the low-carbohydrate craze. The phrase "white foods are bad" is an oversimplification and a source of confusion. While originally the intent of this phrase was related to avoiding refined grains, many have taken it literally over the years and avoided good-for-you white foods that are part of a healthy eating pattern—such as low-fat milk or yogurt, white beans, onions, cauliflower, and bananas.

Takeaway: Just because information is on the Internet does not mean it's true. Ask yourself the questions in "Internet Insight" on page 198 and talk to your health-care team.

The following websites provide valuable and reliable information about diabetes and healthy eating:

DIABETES

American Diabetes Association
www.diabetes.org

JDRF (formerly Juvenile Diabetes Research Foundation)
www.jdrf.org

National Diabetes Education Program (NDEP)
www.ndep.nih.gov

National Institutes of Health—MedlinePlus
www.nlm.nih.gov

HEALTHY EATING

Academy of Nutrition and Dietetics
www.eatright.org

ChooseMyPlate (USDA)
www.choosemyplate.gov

Dietary Guidelines for Americans
www.health.gov/dietaryguidelines

United States Department of Agriculture (USDA) Food and Nutrition Information Center
http://fnic.nal.usda.gov

Reach Out to Others

Reach Out to Your Diabetes Health-Care Team

If you have questions or concerns about diabetes, your meal plan, or other aspects of treatment, ask your diabetes health-care team. Your health-care provider and diabetes educator are dedicated to helping you take an active role in caring for your diabetes.

Reach Out to Family and Friends

People who have a strong support system in place tend to be healthier and recover more quickly from illnesses. Many of the healthy-eating principles you are following to control your diabetes are good for your family as well, making it easier for them to join you in support.

Oftentimes family and friends want to help but don't understand diabetes or know exactly how to offer help. They may seem more like the diabetes police than a diabetes partner. It may help for you to share the "dos and don'ts" from "Diabetes Etiquette for People Who DON'T Have Diabetes" on page 201.

Reach Out to Others with Diabetes

In time, you may be ready to widen your support network by joining a support group, participating in a diabetes class, or connecting with others in the vibrant online diabetes community. The American Diabetes Association even has an online message board that allows people with diabetes to share their ideas, questions, and opinions on a variety of topics. These settings provide great opportunities to discuss common problems and concerns as well as share helpful advice, offer support, and celebrate success in diabetes self-care. Another great way to reach out is to participate in an organized activity that focuses on diabetes, such as a walk, bike ride, or health fair. This can be a fun way for you to make a difference in your local community by raising awareness or raising money for the research and treatment of diabetes. Remember, there is strength in numbers. You are not alone on your journey with diabetes!

Choices, Control, Consequences

Although it would be nice to turn your diabetes eating challenges over to an all-knowing nutrition guru, the fact is that you make the choices every day that have the greatest impact on your health and well-being. Choosing to skip a milkshake in favor of water or another calorie-free drink will certainly affect your diabetes control. No matter how much your doctor or RD/RDN educates you about the benefits of broiling, only you can decide whether fried chicken ends up on your plate. And that's only fair, because you are the one who reaps the rewards of your decisions.

What Do I Eat Now? has presented you with the nutrition strategies and targets you need to live a healthy life with diabetes. You are in control of your choices. Make those choices wisely in order to take the next step on the road to successful self-management!

Diabetes Etiquette for People Who DON'T Have Diabetes

Here's what you can say:

1. DON'T offer unsolicited advice about my eating or other aspects of diabetes. You may mean well, but giving advice about someone's personal habits, especially when it is not requested, isn't very nice. Besides, many of the popularly held beliefs about diabetes ("you should just stop eating sugar") are out of date or just plain wrong.

2. DO realize and appreciate that diabetes is hard work. Diabetes management is a full-time job that I didn't apply for, didn't want and can't quit. It involves thinking about what, when and how much I eat, while also factoring in exercise, medication, stress, blood glucose monitoring and so much more—each and every day.

3. DON'T tell me horror stories about your grandmother or other people with diabetes you have heard about. Diabetes is scary enough and stories like these are not reassuring! Besides, we now know that with good management, odds are good that I can live a long, healthy and happy life with diabetes.

4. DO offer to join me in making healthy lifestyle changes. Not having to be alone with efforts to change, like starting an exercise program, is one of the most powerful ways that you can be helpful. After all, healthy lifestyle changes can benefit everyone!

5. DON'T look so horrified when I check my blood glucose or give myself an injection. It is not a lot of fun for me either. Checking blood glucose and taking medications are things I must do to manage diabetes well. If I have to hide while I do so, it makes it much harder for me.

6. DO ask how you might be helpful. If you want to be supportive, there may be lots of little things I would probably appreciate your help with. However, what I really need may be very different than what you think I need, so please ask first.

7. DON'T offer thoughtless reassurances. When you first learn about my diabetes, you may want to reassure me by saying things like, "Hey, it could be worse; you could have cancer!" This won't make me feel better. And the implicit message seems to be that diabetes is no big deal. However, diabetes (like cancer) IS a big deal.

8. DO be supportive of my efforts for self-care. Help me set up an environment for success by supporting healthy food choices. Please honor my decision to decline a particular food even when you really want me to try it. You are most helpful when you are not being a source of unnecessary temptation.

9. DON'T peek at or comment on my blood glucose numbers without asking me first. These numbers are private unless I choose to share them. It is normal to have numbers that are sometimes too low or too high. Your unsolicited comments about these numbers can add to the disappointment, frustration and anger I already feel.

10. DO offer your love and encouragement. As I work hard to manage diabetes successfully, sometimes just knowing that you care can be very helpful and motivating.

Reprinted with permission from Behavioral Diabetes Institute.[2]

Next Steps

- Think of a situation in which you may be/may have been tempted to overeat. Make a plan for what you'll do when you find yourself in this situation again (because you will at some point).
- Learn more about a diabetes or healthy-eating topic that is of special interest to you; for example, nutrition for athletes with diabetes or vegetarian cooking.
- Call your local chapter of the American Diabetes Association, or check out their website (www.diabetes.org), to find out about activities in your area.

---

[2]Behavioral Diabetes Institute. *Diabetes Etiquette for People Who Don't Have Diabetes.* Available from http://www. behavioraldiabetes.org

What Do I Eat for Dinner?

FOR 45–60 GRAMS OF CARBOHYDRATE*

3 ounces grilled fish

1 cup steamed broccoli and carrots

Spinach salad with 1 tablespoon olive oil
  vinaigrette

1 small slice french bread

6 ounces plain low-fat or fat-free greek yogurt
  with 3/4 cup blueberries and a sprinkling
  of walnuts

Recipes: Lemony Spa Water (8 ounces) or
  Watermelon Rosemary Refresher
  (8 ounces)

FOR 60–75 GRAMS OF CARBOHYDRATE*

3 ounces grilled fish

1/3 cup steamed brown rice

1 cup steamed broccoli and carrots

Spinach salad with 1 tablespoon olive oil
  vinaigrette

1 small slice french bread

6 ounces plain low-fat or fat-free greek yogurt
  with 3/4 cup blueberries and a sprinkling
  of walnuts

Recipes: Lemony Spa Water (8 ounces) or
  Watermelon Rosemary Refresher
  (8 ounces)

For most women, 45–60 grams of carbohydrate at a meal is a good starting point; for most men, 60–75 grams of carbohydrate per meal is appropriate. Check with your diabetes health-care team to find the amount of carbohydrate that's right for you.

Swift, Simple Tips

- Find ready-to-steam broccoli and carrots in either the produce or frozen food section of the grocery store.
- Use bagged, prewashed spinach leaves and a high-quality bottled salad dressing to save some time.
- Use boil-in-bag brown rice, which cooks in just 10 minutes.

LEMONY SPA WATER

SERVES: 8

SERVING SIZE: 8 ounces

PREPARATION TIME: 5 minutes

CHILLING TIME: 2–4 hours

INGREDIENTS

1 lemon, thinly sliced
1/2 cucumber, thinly sliced
1 handful fresh mint
Ice cubes
Water

1. Place lemon and cucumber in a 2-quart pitcher. Gently crush the mint in your hands to release the flavor and aroma, then add to pitcher. Fill pitcher with ice cubes. Add water to the top of the pitcher.
2. Cover and chill for 2–4 hours, then serve. Cover and refrigerate for up to 3 days.

CHOICES/EXCHANGES	BASIC NUTRITIONAL VALUES			
Free Food	**Calories**	0	**Potassium**	0 mg
	Calories from Fat	0	**Total Carbohydrate**	0 g
	Total Fat	0.0 g	Dietary Fiber	0 g
	Saturated Fat	0.0 g	Sugars	0 g
	Trans Fat	0.0 g	**Protein**	0 g
	Cholesterol	0 mg	**Phosphorus**	0 mg
	Sodium	10 mg		

WATERMELON ROSEMARY REFRESHER

SERVES: 8

SERVING SIZE: 8 ounces

PREPARATION TIME: 5 minutes

CHILLING TIME: 2–4 hours

INGREDIENTS

2 cups cubed watermelon

1 sprig fresh rosemary

Ice cubes

Water

1. Place watermelon in a 2-quart pitcher. Gently crush the rosemary in your hands to release the flavor and aroma, then add to pitcher. Fill pitcher with ice cubes. Add water to the top of the pitcher.
2. Cover and chill for 2–4 hours, then serve. Cover and refrigerate for up to 3 days.

Infused Water Tips

Are you trying to find a substitute for sugary sodas or carb-containing fruit juices? Do you want to cut back on diet drinks or bottled "healthy" waters flavored with artificial sweeteners? The subtle flavor of infused water may be just what you're looking for.

Infused waters are simply water with the added bonus of flavor from fruits, vegetables, and herbs. They're easy to prepare and can help you reach a healthy goal of drinking at least eight 8-ounce glasses of fluid each day. Water supports all of our body's functions and we know it's especially important to avoid dehydration if you have diabetes.

We've given you two starter recipes, but feel free to have fun and make your own creative combinations such as:

- Lime or orange slices and mint
- Lemon, lime, and tangerine slices
- Orange slices and cranberries
- Lime slices and raspberries
- Blackberries and sage
- Pineapple chunks and mint
- Cucumber and lime slices
- Key lime or orange slices and a scraped vanilla bean

Chilled infused water served in a clear glass pitcher or mason jar will add a colorful and healthy touch to your table the next time you entertain!

CHOICES/EXCHANGES

Free Food

BASIC NUTRITIONAL VALUES

Calories	10	**Potassium**	45 mg
Calories from Fat	0	**Total Carbohydrate**	3 g
Total Fat	0.0 g	Dietary Fiber	0 g
Saturated Fat	0.0 g	Sugars	2 g
Trans Fat	0.0 g	**Protein**	0 g
Cholesterol	0 mg	**Phosphorus**	0 mg
Sodium	10 mg		

Food for Thought

- *You* are the manager of your diabetes meal plan.
- Continue to learn all you can about diabetes and healthy eating.
- Reach out to others for help and support.

Note: Page numbers followed by *t* refer to tables. Page numbers in **bold** indicate an in-depth discussion.

Metric Equivalents

Liquid Measurement	Metric equivalent
1 teaspoon	5 mL
1 tablespoon *or* 1/2 fluid ounce	15 mL
1 fluid ounce *or* 1/8 cup	30 mL
1/4 cup *or* 2 fluid ounces	60 mL
1/3 cup	80 mL
1/2 cup *or* 4 fluid ounces	120 mL
2/3 cup	160 mL
3/4 cup *or* 6 fluid ounces	180 mL
1 cup *or* 8 fluid ounces *or* 1/2 pint	240 mL
1 1/2 cups *or* 12 fluid ounces	350 mL
2 cups *or* 1 pint *or* 16 fluid ounces	475 mL
3 cups *or* 1 1/2 pints	700 mL
4 cups *or* 2 pints *or* 1 quart	950 mL
4 quarts *or* 1 gallon	3.8 L

Weight Measurement	Metric equivalent
1 ounce	28 g
4 ounces *or* 1/4 pound	113 g
1/3 pound	150 g
8 ounces *or* 1/2 pound	230 g
2/3 pound	300 g
12 ounces *or* 3/4 pound	340 g
1 pound *or* 16 ounces	450 g
2 pounds	900 g

Dry Measurements	Metric equivalent
1 teaspoon	5 g
1 tablespoon	14 g
1/4 cup	57 g
1/2 cup	113 g
3/4 cup	168 g
1 cup	224 g

Length	Metric equivalent
1/8 inch	3 mm
1/4 inch	6 mm
1/2 inch	13 mm
3/4 inch	19 mm
1 inch	2.5 cm
2 inches	5 cm

Fahrenheit	Celsius	Fahrenheit	Celsius
275ºF	140ºC	400ºF	200ºC
300ºF	150ºC	425ºF	220ºC
325ºF	165ºC	450ºF	230ºC
350ºF	180ºC	475ºF	240ºC
375ºF	190ºC	500ºF	260ºC

Weights of common ingredients in grams

Ingredient	1 cup	3/4 cup	2/3 cup	1/2 cup	1/3 cup	1/4 cup	2 Tbsp
Flour, all-purpose (wheat)	120 g	90 g	80 g	60 g	40 g	30 g	15 g
Flour, well-sifted, all-purpose (wheat)	110 g	80 g	70 g	55 g	35 g	27 g	13 g
Sugar, granulated cane	200 g	150 g	130 g	100 g	65 g	50 g	25 g
Confectioner's sugar (cane)	100 g	75 g	70 g	50 g	35 g	25 g	13 g
Brown sugar, packed firmly	180 g	135 g	120 g	90 g	60 g	45 g	23 g
Cornmeal	160 g	120 g	100 g	80 g	50 g	40 g	20 g
Cornstarch	120 g	90 g	80 g	60 g	40 g	30 g	15 g
Rice, uncooked	190 g	140 g	125 g	95 g	65 g	48 g	24 g
Macaroni, uncooked	140 g	100 g	90 g	70 g	45 g	35 g	17 g
Couscous, uncooked	180 g	135 g	120 g	90 g	60 g	45 g	22 g
Oats, uncooked, quick	90 g	65 g	60 g	45 g	30 g	22 g	11 g
Table salt	300 g	230 g	200 g	150 g	100 g	75 g	40 g
Butter	240 g	180 g	160 g	120 g	80 g	60 g	30 g
Vegetable shortening	190 g	140 g	125 g	95 g	65 g	48 g	24 g
Chopped fruits and vegetables	150 g	110 g	100 g	75 g	50 g	40 g	20 g
Nuts, chopped	150 g	110 g	100 g	75 g	50 g	40 g	20 g
Nuts, ground	120 g	90 g	80 g	60 g	40 g	30 g	15 g
Bread crumbs, fresh, loosely packed	60 g	45 g	40 g	30 g	20 g	15 g	8 g
Bread crumbs, dry	150 g	110 g	100 g	75 g	50 g	40 g	20 g
Parmesan cheese, grated	90 g	65 g	60 g	45 g	30 g	22 g	11 g